WALKING

with FAY

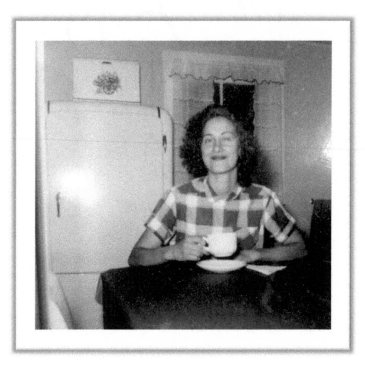

~ Fay, circa 1952 ~

WALKING

with FAY

My Mother's
Uncharted Path
into Dementia

CAROLYN BIRRELL

atmosphere press

This book is a memoir. It reflects the author's present recollections of experiences over time. Some names have been changed, some events have been compressed, and some dialogue has been recreated.

CONTENTS

To my mother.

You wouldn't have liked the attention, and certainly not the content, but you would've loved me.

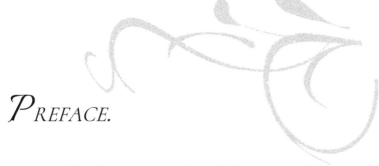

$\mathcal{P}$REFACE.

In 2012, I flew down to Georgia to kidnap my mother.

She'd been showing escalating signs of early-stage dementia for some time, but I'd become good at dismissing each one as signs of getting old. It was the calls from her local sheriff and the Department of Family Services that finally moved me to action.

My plan was to trick her into thinking she was spending the summer with me in North Idaho. I would purchase a house near me, fill it with her personal things to make it look like her home in Georgia, and keep a gentle eye on her from a close distance.

Dementia is tricky, though. Until it progresses to its more advanced stages, those affected sound perfectly reasonable most of the time. They carry on conversations with strangers and seem quite normal. They invent stories that are dreadful but sound believable. They can grocery shop, drive a car, and cook for themselves. And they can certainly walk out any door you try to secure them safely behind.

My mother was all of these things. And she was a walker, literally and figuratively. In the literal sense, she was up and out as soon as the sun came up, and sometimes again after it set. Figuratively, her ever-changing behaviors made it impossible for me to keep up, and if by chance I did, she switched direction and was gone again, always leaving me one step behind.

This is the story of my mother, her dementia, and our struggles to navigate her journey together. My hope is that it will help those who are drowning like I was; the sons, daughters, and loved ones who find themselves dealing with this sneaky, debilitating disease that not only robs the person you love of their mental faculties, but effectively changes them into someone you struggle to recognize, let alone like.

It's filled with all the things I needed back then. I needed to see that there were others just like me who felt lost, overwhelmed, and scared to death, frankly. I needed validation that I was doing the best thing for my mother even while she pummeled me with accusations of abuse. I needed confirmation that my decisions and actions were those of a good daughter, even when they felt like a betrayal. I needed to know that the mistakes I made along the way were the same as those made by others in my place; and I especially needed reassurance that my feelings of guilt, grief, and even anger were normal as the mother I knew and loved vanished before me in slow motion.

Believe me, you're not alone on this new, scary path you're traveling.

Your loved one may not force feed stuffed animals vanilla pudding or burn their neighbor's mail like my mother did, but my hope is that those of you who are living through the sad realities of your loved one's slow and tortuous farewell will find solace as you deal with it realistically and with a heart at peace.

SHE WAS JUST GETTING OLD.

Year One – Stage 2
(Age Associated Memory Impairment)

"Morning ma'am, this is Lieutenant Davey from Franklin County Sheriff's Department. I'm calling about your mother."

It was 5am Idaho time, too early for my alarm clock and birds, really. The room was black, and I'd just been jarred awake by the insistent shrill of my phone, setting every nerve in my body on high alert.

"We're real worried about her. Been getting calls about her driving on the wrong side of the road, cuttin' people off, that sort a thing." He began recounting each of the complaints he'd recently received as I blinked my eyes into focus and forced myself to concentrate.

I cleared my throat, *"Well, could you pull her over next time? Maybe give her a ticket? Can you take away her license or something?"*

"No ma'am. Can't do that until I see her do it myself. I was hopin' you could talk to her."

Talk to her? I lived 3,000 miles away from my mother's rural north Georgia town where she lived by herself, a fiercely independent and very proud 79-year-old. I knew exactly how that call from me would be received. *"Hey Mom, I heard you've been driving erratically these days. Seems you're causing a lot of concern around town. Maybe it's time to give up your driver's license. Where did I hear that? Oh, from your town sheriff – who heard it from your friends and neighbors."* It took

3

me three short seconds to consider the repercussions of making a call like that, leaving no doubt in my mind that things were just going to have to work themselves out without my help.

I thanked the lieutenant, took his number, and promised to broach the subject with my mother, which I absolutely did *not* do later that morning during our daily phone call.

My mom and dad moved to Georgia after my dad retired from a life of plumbing in western New York where I was raised. Their house was paid off and their three kids were grown. They were entering their golden years, but New York state property taxes and astronomical winter heating bills made it hard to budget on Dad's modest Social Security checks. I'd been living in Atlanta for several years and reporting back to them how much I loved it, so after a few holiday visits (they couldn't believe they were wearing t-shirts in the backyard on Christmas morning!), they focused their attentions south.

They found their perfect little house – a brick rancher in North Georgia, *"Not too close to that big city you moved to,"* on a country acre just a couple hours' drive from me. It was 1992. Their new town boasted a hospital, grocery store, and a dozen churches. Dad tinkered in his wood shop out back and Mom packed her garden with vegetables. They planted two fig trees and were busy making friends in their new congregation. They marveled at the azaleas in bloom each spring when they expected snow. And just eight years later, Dad became sick and died, leaving Mom suddenly alone.

Overnight, I became "Keeper of the Mother," managing Saturday trips to her house while trying to live my own life two hours away. My sister Roxanne still lived in New York and could only manage annual visits, and even though my brother Dale lived in Atlanta near me, he was never short of reasons why he rarely made a trip to see her. I was 35, a busy real estate agent partnered with my husband, Sam, and ill prepared to take on my new post.

The full day it took to drive there, visit, and circle back home didn't leave much to the weekend, and the balancing act was grueling. We'd make an early start of it, Sam driving and me with a stack of client files on my lap, making phone calls. We'd try not to rush through lunch and then begin hinting it was time to leave around 3pm. By the time we pulled into our driveway, the day was over and we each felt it.

Maybe she didn't need me to drop in on her every week, and maybe I made more of it than was needed, but I went. A missed Saturday left me squarely seated between relief and anxiety. I needed the break, but I anguished over the image I easily conjured of my mother wandering through every room in her house, alone and missing her family.

Mom did seem to bounce back quickly after Dad died. Happier, maybe; liberated from forty-five years of cooking and cleaning for a husband she didn't do much with anymore but bicker. Our daily phone calls were filled with stories of her working in her garden and sharing tomatoes with friends. A stray cat had shown up recently and made his home in her carport. She named him Ghost. He was an excellent mouser, and his daily escapades became a regular topic of conversation. She'd started going back to church and recounted all the goings-on of her neighbors she spotted during her morning walks. She never missed a day, not even when it rained. *"That's what umbrellas are for."*

Sam and I had been playing with the idea of leaving the city and simplifying our lives a few years before my father passed away. We were flying high above the real estate bubble of the 90s and the frenetic lifestyle we'd created for ourselves was taking its toll on our marriage. We'd even started looking at properties in rural areas of the northwest that were close enough to culture and entertainment yet still buffered from a crazy-large population like Atlanta.

Those plans ground to a halt when my dad died. How could I announce to my mother that I was thinking about leaving her alone so soon afterward? I couldn't imagine how she'd survive on her own without us nearby to swoop in and handle things when she needed, so we shelved that dream and let a few more years pass.

That time came, though, and I remember the day I told her we were moving. We'd stumbled upon a piece of property in North Idaho on the internet, flew out to take a look, and instantly fell in love with the area. After several more scouting trips disguised as vacations, we decided it was time to head out West. All I had to do was tell Fay.

I drove to her house by myself that weekend to deliver the news. She was my mother and she was alone, so I wanted to proceed as gently with her as I could. Visions of tears and pleas to stay had been in my head the entire drive there, and I was filled with dread by the time I pulled into her driveway. She surprised me, though. She let me finish my well-rehearsed monologue about how over-worked we were, how dangerously stressed our marriage was from the amount of business we took on, and how we envisioned a slower pace in the beautiful mountain region of the great Northwest. She didn't seem the least bit upset or anxious that her youngest, closest daughter was deserting her.

She'd be fine, she said. She had her church and her friends. She was content. *"Go to Idaho."* I left her that day with my mind in a fog. I'd worked myself up for a terrible confrontation and instead I pulled out of her driveway with full consent and a to-go container of leftovers. I replayed our conversation on the drive home and reassured myself she was well-adjusted and capable, but my guilt and apprehension were in full swing. It crushed me to leave her behind, but that day came, and I did leave.

The distance between us didn't feel as vast as I'd anticipated, and we developed a comfortable routine almost immediately. She'd get in from her morning walks and watch the clock until it struck 10am to dial me. Her calls became my 7am alarm, beginning with tales from her most recent walking escapade as I shuffled into the kitchen to grind beans in spurts so I wouldn't drown her out. Then, settled on the couch with a cup of coffee in my lap, we'd fill an hour with any number of topics. I don't remember exactly when I began noticing her story loops, but I do remember how I responded.

"Mom! How many times are you going to repeat that same story about your bank teller? You've told it to me three times in this conversation!"

She never missed a beat when I brought it to her attention, countering, *"I know I did, but it was funny!"* And she never seemed hurt by my retort. I'd hang up feeling a little unsettled, not as much by the impatience I hadn't yet learned to temper, but more the fact that this was happening in the first place. And then I'd just as quickly remind myself she was only getting quirky. It was 2006, and little did I know then, this was just the beginning of a long span of years I was about to embark on with my mother.

I'd laugh about it with friends, and we'd joke that we could tell we were getting old by the way we'd begun comparing the bizarre things our parents did. The thought of dementia truly never occurred to me. Her stories were more like tracks set on repeat every two or three minutes. *She was just getting old.* She'd tell me about the pan of lasagna she made for Jerry, her neighbor whose wife left him. She talked about her daily walks and the woman who waved to her from the window whenever she passed her house down the street – a single mother who had her hands full raising two kids by herself who should just find herself a good man to take care of her. She may have retold these stories half a dozen times in one call, and it may have driven me crazy, but I held tight to my belief that *she was only doing what all seniors do.*

It wasn't until she started mentioning the man at the end of the driveway who was watching her house at night that I knew I had to stop pretending everything was fine. She said she knew he'd been there from the cigarette butts she found every morning when she headed out on her walk and swore she counted a few more each day. And that marked a point on the timeline when my mother's curious personality changes began to worsen.

YOU CAN'T WRAP THEM IN A STRAITJACKET AND BRING THEM WHERE YOU WANT THEM.

I didn't wait long after settling into our new home in Idaho before I began hinting to my mom that she might like to move closer to me. I started sending her clippings from the local newspaper and endless photos I took to show her how beautiful it was where we lived. I kept at it for a full year. She loved to hear the stories, but she was unbending in her responses. *"It's out of the question. Why would I leave my home and everyone I know? Leave my church? What would happen to my garden? Ghost! I'd have no friends! And how would Roxanne visit if I moved so far away? What about Dale?"*

My pleas to have her near me became increasingly more insistent over time, and I began to lose patience with her countless reasons not to come to Idaho. With every sure excuse she delivered, my feelings became that much more bruised. I missed her. I wanted her with me, and her unusual new behaviors were becoming harder to push to the edges of my mind.

I was already feeling pretty beat up over Mom's ready rejections to my invitations, but the heaviest blow came one afternoon after receiving a call from her pastor asking if my mother was ill. *"We haven't seen her in church in over a year and we're worried about her."* My head spun as I replayed our morning calls, many centered on her elaborately staged narratives about her congregation. She could recite attendance, hymns she sang, and even the pastor's latest sermon. It was all fabricated? One of her weightiest reasons not to move closer to me had just been blown out of the water, and I didn't know what to do with that.

I thanked the pastor for calling, assured him that she was well, and that I'd do what I could to encourage her to rejoin them next Sunday. No, I didn't think she needed the van (well, she probably did, but convincing *her* of that...). And no, I was sure it wasn't anything anyone had said at church to put her off.

I decided to investigate and made a few calls of my own. I was shocked when I learned from her neighbor across the street that Mom's garden was a thatched mess and hadn't produced a vegetable in ages. That story about sharing tomatoes with her friends was born from pure imagination. And knowing that she was lucky to receive a visit from Roxanne and Dale once a year left me with the realization, imagined or otherwise, that it wasn't their regular visits she was worried about missing, my mother just didn't care enough to be near me! She'd simply rather be in her house by herself, no church, no garden, no Carolyn.

Did I confront her? No. What was I going to do with the truth, anyway? Chastise her? These lies about church and her non-existent garden were so outlandish to me that they didn't seem possible. And acknowledging them would only make this thing real, so I ignored it. But I couldn't let it go either, so I came in from another direction and resolved to change my mother's mind instead. I would introduce her to my charming town and show her its beauty in person.

I began with the offer of an all-expenses-paid trip to Idaho. It was our second summer there and she finally agreed to let me fly her out for a visit. I surprised her by bringing my Aunt Jack, one of her last three surviving sisters, out from Portland, too. They hadn't seen each other in over a decade, and their shrill exclamations and dramatic embraces prompted dozens of smiles and comments at the baggage claim. They were like giddy schoolgirls their entire trip.

Surely she'd realize how nice it was to have me and her sister close by on a permanent basis. I promised to bring Aunt Jack here or put Mom on the short flight there as often as she wanted, and I'd do the same for Roxanne. By moving to Idaho, I explained, she'd actually see everyone much more than she does now, especially me.

I could squeeze that pitch into any conversation, and I practiced it daily.

"See Mom? We could go out for breakfast all the time if you lived here."

"There must be twenty churches to choose from in my town!"

"You could have a beautiful garden here and I'd have it tilled for you every spring."

I was always met with a bobbing head and fixed smile. Just enough to show me she heard me, but zero commitment.

I crammed every sort of adventure into their visit. We drove the six-mile loop through the Wildlife Refuge with Mom and Aunt Jack on inner tubes in the bed of my truck so they could *"be closer to the deer and moose if we see any."* We gambled at the casino, each of them protesting, *"What ever happened to the one-armed bandits??! How are we supposed to work these new push-button things?!"* every few minutes, and too loudly. We picnicked at the river. They tasted elk steaks for the first time. They SAW elk for the first time. We went for a horse drawn buggy ride through town and out to the Indian reservation where they exclaimed (also too loudly), *"We haven't seen real Indians since we played with them as kids in Kansas!"*

We rode the chairlift up the side of Schweitzer Mountain where it was *"too COLD and too WINDY."* Mom fell asleep on the return ride down and Aunt Jack lost her shoe down into the ravine. I took them to Three Mile Antique Mall just north of town where I could hear my mother exclaiming, *"I have that!"* and *"I have three of those!"* at booth after booth throughout the mall.

Even Sam, my newly ex-husband, contributed to their good time. *"A shame you two divorced; he was so nice to us, and now you'll NEVER find a husband in such a small town,"* they said (in unison and with a little too much conviction). He took them for a picnic and four-wheeler ride perched atop bales of hay around his farm. Sam's rooster, Buddy, rode along. I think that day was the highlight of their trip.

Their seven-day visit ended with a drive to the airport and kisses and hugs at the entrance, but no promises from Fay to see me again soon or of wishing she could stay.

But I never stopped trying. I continued to send photos and always had a new adventure to tell her about during our phone calls. I cajoled, tempted, even teased her that I'd find her a new husband with all the old cowboys we had in our town. I reasoned with her that Roxanne only saw her once a year, and Dale may live close by, but he hardly ever visited. In my eyes, there was no reason for her to stay in Georgia with no one to take her to her doctor's appointments, *"Who needs a doctor, anyway,"* drive her to the grocery store, *"I can drive myself,"* or mow her lawn, *"What they charge to mow! I'll do it myself,"* which she didn't.

Her new favorite line was she didn't want to live with her daughter and be a burden, so I told her I'd buy her a house instead. The conversation would stop, and all I could hear was her breathing on the other end of the line as I imagined her brain winding up for her next serve. There simply wasn't anything I could say to convince her to come. She was "with it" enough to say, *"Absolutely not,"* and where did that leave me? You can't wrap them in a straitjacket and bring them where you want them, and even if I did go kidnap her, she was perfectly able to remove herself from any living arrangement I created for her. At least that's what I still thought, so I decided to just wait until she couldn't make that decision on her own and hope nothing catastrophic happened in the meantime.

It still amazes me when I reflect on all the things I let slide. I see it so clearly now, when talking with people who are beginning to "notice things" about their parents/loved ones/friends. We all see what we want to see, and only that. We practice overlooking the rest until something monumental happens and forces us to shine a light on it. I became skilled at self-deception, and I could out-reason every one of my mother's newfound idiosyncrasies. Until I couldn't.

Shortly after my mother returned to Georgia from her trip, my brother called, demanding, *"Just what is it you're planning to do with Mom's house and all her money?"*

First, know that I might receive a phone call from Dale twice a year, and one of those is on my birthday, so this call had to be pretty important. Second, Mom had no money. He pressed on, recounting to me his conversation with her after she got back from Idaho. She'd told him she was certain his sister (that would be me) was trying to get her to move out West so she could sell her house out from under her and take all her money. And without waiting for my response, he asked me again what I planned to do with the proceeds.

Good Great Lord, really?

This was how she interpreted my efforts to arrange her exciting trip, see her sister for the first time in forever, and our wonderful time together in general? His words ping ponged around my brain as I tried to form words. Wait, what?! What's this sudden commitment of his to my mother's well-being? Dale's thrice-a-year visits to Mom's were predictable events by now. They included two loads of dirty laundry to wash and fold, a homecooked meal with leftovers to take home, and if he was lucky, a check to help with rent.

It was certainly not the sort of thing *my* mother would ever say about her youngest, the one who stayed closest to her and asked for nothing. It was just another thwack on the head I should have noticed to help me focus on what was really going on with her. I can read this now with total astonishment at the depth of my denial back then. I had actually called my mother quirky! I rolled my eyes about her funny little antics and how she was getting old *"right in front of me."* I regaled my friends with tales of her new and strange behaviors, but I didn't truly acknowledge what was happening to her.

My now annual trips to Georgia and our morning calls were my only options left if she refused to come to me. I told myself they were going to have to be enough for me to keep an eye on her for now. And of course, it turns out they weren't. Even as every visit to her house hatched a new series of nagging concerns, I methodically pushed them to the corners of my brain. Things didn't seem right there, but *that was just my unpredictable, aging mother.*

I still remember my last visit to her house. I'd arrived late at night after a long day of cross-country travel and connecting flights and was looking for anything to eat besides airport food. She was delighted to see me and ushered me into the kitchen to find something left over from dinner to reheat. When she flipped the light switch, I was greeted by a kitchen with counters I knew were there but couldn't see. There wasn't one bare spot to simply make a sandwich. Used paper plates were stacked and leaning against the coffee pot, threatening to topple over. Empty prescription bottles, *"Good for seeds,"* were scattered among folded bread bags, *"Handy storage."* There were so many dirty coffee cups that I thought she'd just had a group of ladies over for Bunco, but she didn't play the game and she never had people over.

Spoiling tomatoes lined her windowsill, fruit flies busily landing and launching from their oozing spots. A trail of ants weaved a crooked line to the weeping butter in a dish she insisted be kept at room temperature, *"Otherwise it'll tear the bread."* She opened the solid packed refrigerator and food in varying stages of decomposition tumbled out onto her feet. The sour smell of decay that wafted out of it was so offensive that it sent me scrambling to open the door to the carport so I could air out the room.

I poured myself a bowl of stale Cheerios and sniffed the milk before using it.

If you're thinking, *"Well, concerned daughter, why didn't you disinfect her kitchen? Throw away those tomatoes! Clear out that fridge!"* I'd have a ready explanation. My mother raised me to be the good daughter who does what she's told to do or not to do. I was told *not* to touch anything. I was even warned not to go after the ants. *"It's useless. I've tried everything. They'll come right back,"* she snapped.

I didn't clean one thing under her watchful eyes during my stay. I didn't organize her papers or throw away her empty cans. The only way to use the bathroom was to lock myself inside and scrub the grime as quickly and quietly as I could. Within minutes she'd be rapping on the door, *"You'd better not be moving anything around in there. I know what you're doing!"*

And just like that, my four-day visit was over, and it was time to pack my suitcase and scurry off to the airport. I'd done my duty and was released until my next visit, returning home with plenty of goofy Fay stories to tell Robert (that unlikely new boyfriend I'd managed to meet in my "small town") and the girls in my 8am step class.

There's no doubt I didn't want to even hazard a guess at some deeper problem – *what I wanted was for everything to quit feeling so weird and return to the way I remembered it.* I didn't like her new housekeeping style that differed so dramatically from that of the tidy mother who raised me to make my bed every morning or play with new toys only after the old ones had been put away. Her story loops drove me crazy, and her new habit of assuming the worst of everyone from her hairdresser, store clerk, and even her elderly neighbor was painful to listen to.

But when I looked at her, I still saw my mom, maybe just a little grayer and a bit more wrinkled. Who cared if she did burn the bacon now, and her milk curdled my watery coffee every morning I was there? Hadn't she earned the right by now to adopt some of the idiosyncrasies that come with aging? And if she wouldn't let me throw away the spoiled carton of milk when I brought in a new one from the Super Saver because *we could use it for something,*" so what? I told myself those were just random little hiccups on my trip – she still seemed "okay." In fact, she insisted she was, and that declaration settled comfortably in my head. I had a busy life to return to with no room for figuring out the confusing needs of this new version of my mother that I really wasn't ready or willing to accept anyway.

So off I'd go, back home and pleased with myself for fulfilling my daughterly duties. I'd just spent four uneasy days with my aging, difficult mother, trying not to piss her off by telling her what to do, and unable to fix all the little things I could see needed fixing.

You must think I really am crazy.

My regular morning calls with my mother resumed, but they had begun to change, too. Some mornings were uneventful, but more often, I could detect an underlying current of tension in her voice. She seemed nervous and distracted, her tone was higher, and her words came faster, leaving little room for two-way conversation. Those were the days I'd learned to brace myself for some new story that would become progressively more alarming. And each one seemed more bizarre than the last.

Her tone would become sharper as she elaborated for me some scenario in which she'd been wronged, simply beside herself with shock and rage. She'd shriek into the receiver that every one of her magazines and Grandma's prized quilts had been scattered all over the house during the night while she slept. She knew exactly who the culprit was, too: the lady from the bank. That lady had her eye on those quilts ever since she'd brought one in to show her. And the magazines – well, that woman was enough of a lunatic and spiteful besides, to rearrange them all while she was there. Someone was even getting into her bank account and paying her bills for her!

When the "incidents" first began, I'd attempt to reason with her, asking why the lady from the bank didn't just take the quilts home with her if she liked them so much. I'd challenge her with, *"Why take the trouble to break in just to move them around?"* Without missing a beat, my mother would angrily retort that she knew I was trying to make her sound crazy and why did I always have to question everything she told me? We'd do this dance for weeks. Every. Day. For weeks.

No amount of rationalizing or reassuring would do, until I finally thought to offer having her locks changed. She was thrilled to have the locksmith out, but once her new locks were installed, she refused to hand over her now-defunct set of keys, *"And give the locksmith a way to get inside my house? You must think I really am crazy."* Now armed with a key ring filled with a mix of new AND old keys, you might guess how often my mother successfully entered her home. This led to a rash of panicked phone calls over the next several weeks made from any random neighbor's house (since she'd been locked out of her own) that she couldn't get in, because of *"that locksmith who didn't even know how to change a lock."*

So a second call was made to the locksmith, followed by another $150 invoice, to make a repeat trip out to her house for a whole new lock change. This time I was able to convince her on the phone to put all the old keys into a Ziploc baggie and hide them in her closet, *"where no one could find them and use them to break in."* That made perfect sense to her, and I mailed a second check to the locksmith.

I counted two weeks of pleasant calls with no major fires to stamp out and was beginning to think $300 was a small amount to pay for peace.

Then her wedding rings and other jewelry went missing. There was no doubt in her mind that someone was still managing to get in. Our same Lieutenant Davey went by to look around. He called me from her living room to report that he could see no evidence of intrusion. I could hear my mother in the background mimicking his southern accent and saying something about him being incompetent; and yes, we had the locks changed for a third time – adding to her collection of keys in the closet. Marty, the locksmith's owner, finally called me to share his sneaking suspicion that *"Your mother might be going senile."* He told me it pained him to have to charge me again, asked if my address was the same, and about a week later, I sent him my third check.

A few uneventful months went by when one morning my mother called me to tell me her incredible luck – the burglar had returned her jewelry and hidden it in the laundry hamper! She was ecstatic! But she was as equally unconcerned that this burglar had somehow made his way back into her home to return everything. Nor was she perplexed as to why he chose the laundry hamper to return the stolen goods. I was simply happy not to have to schedule a fourth service call with Marty.

If any of this sounds funny to you now, it certainly wasn't to me then. I would question her repeatedly over how she could've possibly lost her jewelry, to which she insisted repeatedly (and sharply) that it had been stolen, to which I repeatedly (and equally sharply) refused to believe. I was impatient with her. I felt forced to listen to every ridiculous detail she gave me during each explanation she manufactured.

I felt hugely inconvenienced each time I had to reschedule the series of appointments *between* each of the locksmith's first, second, and third trip to her house because my mother couldn't remember to stay home and be there to answer the door.

I made sure my mother understood what a hassle this was for me, and how her judgment and truthfulness were now in question. Things I'm not proud to admit, but this wasn't the kind of behavior I'd had any experience with, and especially not with this new mother of mine.

Mine was the honest mom. Growing up in our house, telling lies guaranteed you a soapy mouth. To this day, the smell of Irish Spring triggers my eyes to tear up and my mouth to water, and not in a good way.

No, this version was an impostor. And a troublesome one.

My phone would ring, it would be my mom, and I was guaranteed to have some blazing fire to put out.

These little instances should've been wakeup calls for me; I know that now. Starting with my first call from Lieutenant Davey. I'll admit, even that pre-dawn conversation with him didn't truly alarm me. It was more of an aggravation, really, with him trying to make something my problem when *he* was the law. *He* should've been doing something about it. How could I possibly stop her bad driving? It was easy for me to redirect any concern I may have had into criticism over how he should've handled things. And I found out later that he had tried.

He drove to my mother's house the day after he called me, after all. He tapped on her door and was invited in for coffee. He told her he was worried about her. That the whole town was in fact worried about her (big mistake). I can picture him nervously trying to make his case, stammering over his words like he did with me the previous morning. He described the calls he'd gotten from people reporting her erratic driving (even bigger mistake), at which point she removed his coffee cup from the table, called him a liar and told him to get out of her house. My sweet mother who wouldn't say "poo" if she had a mouthful of it, had just said a mouthful.

No, my wakeup call came about two months later from someone named Mrs. Breem, with the Department of Health and Family Welfare (DHFW). It seems Mom had missed her hair appointment, a wash-and-set she had every Friday without fail, so Miss Janice, her hairdresser, drove around the block to peek in Mom's windows (because that's what good hairdressers do). Seeing her car in the driveway, lights on inside the house and the TV flashing but no Fay, she called the police. They found her on the floor and incoherent, so they rushed her to the hospital. Her blood glucose levels were dangerously high, indicating she'd not taken her diabetes medication with any regularity, if at all. It took several days for them to stabilize her and determine she could leave the hospital, but because she couldn't give a friend's or family member's name to pick her up, they called the DHFW.

Mrs. Breem was assigned to her and carted her home. She was instructed to visit her house every day to check in on her, and it took exactly two visits before Mom refused to come to the door.

"WHAT KIND OF DAUGHTER ARE YOU?"

My call from Mrs. Breem wasn't like Lieutenant Davey's. She wasn't sweet, timid, or nervous. She was abrupt, and she was pissed. Our conversation went along the lines of, *"What kind of daughter would allow her own mother to live in that pig sty she's in, wandering around alone in that dark house all day, drinking chicken stock out of a can with a hole punched in it?"*

"Wait, I was just there! Well, six months ago. Maybe eight. I know she's slipped a little with her housekeeping habits, and she's got this obsession about an intruder. And she's stopped going to church, but still..."

"Your mother is in what we call a crisis state. She's lost 48 pounds between her 6-month doctor checkups – were you aware of that? – and she's missed her last two appointments. Your mother's diabetes prescription expired three months ago. If you don't do something about removing her from this situation, the state will step in and do something about it."

I didn't know what *"do something about it"* was, but I swallowed twice and croaked out something about getting an airline ticket as soon as I was able and flying out there to see what could be done. I don't remember her saying goodbye; I don't remember anything but my total, hot shame. My head was swimming. How could I have missed this? Everything Mrs. Breem told me was everything I'd already witnessed with my own eyes. Maybe not that part about the can of chicken stock. It was as if having someone else state it as fact to me made it real. Like, *"Oh, I guess she really is living in a pig sty with ants and fruit flies and sour milk and rotting who-knows-what in the fridge. And she is my mother. And I am a good daughter, but what good daughter would allow things to get this bad?"*

WE KNEW WE'D HAVE TO (GULP) LIE TO HER.

So what did I do? I immediately dialed my sister to dilute the blame I'd just been assigned by half. To her credit, the first words out of Roxanne's mouth after I finished my story about Mrs. Breem's call were, *"What can I do to help?"* I knew there wasn't much she could do to contribute, but at that moment, her words were everything I needed. I had no idea how to proceed, but at least I knew my burden was going to be shared.

Roxanne is older by a little over a year, and although we aren't separated much by age, we've never had that sisterly kind of closeness. Our parents adopted my brother, sister, and me as babies, a couple of years apart from each other, and I don't remember it being any other way – we were simply siblings.

We were raised together, played together, and suffered under the same house rules, complete with early bedtimes, no dating, and no whistling at the dinner table. We hung out in different groups when we were old enough to choose – Roxanne with the tougher crowd and I with the cheerleaders. She was the one who got caught with the cigarettes and booze while I was the straight A student who somehow managed to never get caught.

We played together when there was no one else and did chores together because we had to. That pretty much guaranteed a good fight here and there.

When Dale was 12 and I was 8, he and some neighbor kids coaxed me into a truck tire inner tube and rolled me down a hill like the Kool Aid commercial. They wanted to be just like the cool kids they saw on TV, and I was the lucky one who fit inside the tube. Everyone shouted, *"Hey Kool Aid!"* as they launched me over the edge. I didn't make it to the bottom like the pretty girl in the commercial did, and instead slammed into the side of a parked camper. They said they heard the "snap" right before my endless shrieking, and when they finally had me standing, crooked arm dangling at my side, they all agreed it was broken.

Our mother was at the hairdresser's getting a perm, and at our age we either didn't know how to or certainly didn't dare call an ambulance. We already knew we were in trouble and didn't want to make it worse by making a decision only adults made. So everyone huddled around me murmuring their apologies while we nervously waited for our mother to get home.

I don't remember much about the trip to the hospital or the punishment Dale received, but I do remember Mom's soft boiled eggs on toast and orange sherbet. He was so sorry that I let him sign my cast first. We didn't play together much after that. Not so much because of the inner tube fiasco, but more because I was still a little girl and he was almost a teen. Maybe the mutual trauma from my broken arm reinforced that. Who knows? True, he was my brother, but there were enough years between us to make our lives seem worlds apart and prevented us from ever being close friends. At least that's how I've always rationalized it.

I wonder if Roxanne remembers the time I put her tooth through her bottom lip with a soup ladle while she washed and I dried. I don't recall why we were fighting, but it likely had to do with the fact that neither of us wanted to dry and one of us was certain to be stuck doing it. Back and forth we'd go, slamming down dishes and spraying water until we were finally screaming at each other. I'd had enough and snatched up the ladle and whacked her. The force of the blow and the shock on her face as blood shot out in every direction stunned me and I was instantly hysterical. I was so distraught over what I'd done that she ended up consoling *me,* promising she wouldn't tell Mom if I would just stop crying (I still would have told if it had been me). We staunched the flow and wiped up the mess with a dish towel that we buried in the trash. That marked a period of truce between us that lasted the rest of our teenage years, but we never developed that close sisterly bond you hear about, and as adults we continued to drift further apart.

There's always been that random phone call, usually tied to a birthday, and although it's never been unpleasant, it would quickly progress to the weather and we were usually saying goodbye within ten minutes. There was no obvious reason why we three kids shouldn't all be a full part of each other's lives, but we just never forged those relationships.

My sister had her own family to keep her busy now – two twenty-something daughters who'd blessed her with six grandkids between them. Her oldest daughter, husband, and four kids were sharing her 2-bedroom apartment while saving for a place of their own. She had a mail carrier route that kept her in a car all day, and no savings earmarked "Aging Mother."

As I recited the call from Lieutenant Davey and Mrs. Breem, we compared notes on our past couple of visits to Mom's and the shambles everything was in. Were we overreacting? I hoped she'd say we were. She didn't.

Should we give it some time? Maybe it's just a phase. Maybe I could convince Mom to let me call someone in to help. We couldn't, it wasn't, and she most certainly wouldn't.

We had to do something, but neither of us knew quite how to begin. Our first stab at a solution came easily enough, though, in the form of our brother Dale. He lived alone in a basement apartment in Atlanta. He was currently unemployed and had recently had his driver's license revoked from getting his third DUI. He'd just sold his car to pay his overdue rent and next month's payment loomed in the distance. It made perfect sense! Dale gets a free place to stay in exchange for being Mom's helper around the house and Mom gets to spend time with her son who never visits. And who knows, maybe our mother's constant presence would curb his drinking binges. We agreed I would call Dale and present this incredible opportunity to him.

The offer landed flatly. I remember asking, *"Are you still there? Hello?"* I pushed on, *"And it'll only be for a little while. And you can have everything. The house, her possessions, everything!"*

"But what'll I DO while I'm out there? She lives two hours outside the city!" he complained.

I explained how he could use the money from the sale of her house and personal things to buy something nice when he returned to Atlanta. He could even have her car. And the whole time he was there, he wouldn't have to pay rent or utilities; even his food would be covered. Did I point out how much it would mean to our mother? Or to Roxanne and me? I did, but it was the tangible terms he revisited with me several times before he agreed. But he agreed.

As unenthusiastic as his acceptance of our offer was, I dialed Roxanne and screamed into the phone, *"He's going to do it! It's going to be perfect! Mom's going to be so happy! I'm calling her now!"*

If Dale's response was flat, my mother's was dead. *"Why would I want Dale to live here with me? I don't need anybody to take care of me. And he drinks!"*

How our mother knew about her son's well-guarded secret was beyond me, but I rebounded quickly and told her how he had to sell his car to pay last month's rent and how he was struggling to make ends meet in the city. Plus, he sounded so incredibly lonely whenever I spoke with him on the phone ("twice a year" didn't need to be mentioned). After another long pause, she said she'd think about it.

Two weeks and nine phone calls later, all parties agreed that Dale would move in with Mom at the end of the month. I ignored the degree of persuasion I'd needed to solidify this arrangement and instead reveled in my relief that our Fay-troubles were over. Visions of Mom and Dale relaxing on the porch, working in the garden, and enjoying Mom's long walks together were so vivid in my mind it was as if they'd already happened and were now just memories to recall. It was the kind of pure you feel when everything seems possible and right.

Roxanne called me three days before the move, *"Have you heard from Dale? I've left him a few messages and Mom hasn't heard from him in a couple of weeks."* My heart sank to the bottom of my rib cage. I dialed him after we hung up. I tried him again that afternoon. I began calling every hour for the next two days. At 2am on what was supposed to be move-in day, my phone rang and I let it go to voicemail until morning. My alarm clock reminded me of my pending message, and I was greeted by Dale's slurred and painfully enunciated explanation to me how he couldn't move to "the country." There'd be nothing for him to do out there and he was sorry. Then silence.

He didn't answer his phone for months after that, and I stopped calling. It didn't matter anymore anyway. Mom seemed to forget the whole thing within a week and never mentioned it again. I was done being mad at him, but I was hugely disappointed and anxious all over again about our mother's uncertain future.

Our morning calls continued to alarm me. She seemed to have an unending supply of nighttime intruders, window peepers, and shifty bank tellers. But as nerve wracking and just plain aggravating as these were to navigate, Mrs. Breem and her promise "to do something" haunted me. We really did need to *do something.*

I'd never stopped lobbying for my mother to move to Idaho, and Roxanne agreed that our job now was to get her there. But how were we going to convince her to move out of her home and all the way across the United States to be closer to me because we didn't think she was capable of living alone any longer? We knew we'd have to (gulp) lie to her.

We grew up in a strictly patriarchal, working-class family. Dinner was on the table thirty minutes after Dad got home, and we were all there to eat it, not talk about it. The proverbial, "Children are to be seen and not heard," was alive and well in our house, and talking back might have crossed our minds like a flash, but we never acted on it. Maybe Roxanne did, once.

As strict as that sounds, ours was the mother who colored vinegary Easter eggs with us and hid our baskets in the yard, even when there was snow. We'd wake up Easter morning and couldn't wait to go find what Peter Cottontail had left for us, fully anticipating the once-a-year solid chocolate rabbit from the local candy maker just outside of town. Then it was off to church in our special Easter clothes and maybe even new white gloves if the girls were lucky. I felt like the prettiest, most loved daughter.

Mom could always be counted on to stop at George's Soft Swirl on the way home from Saturday morning grocery shopping to get a plain vanilla swirl for her and a chocolate twist dip for me. Roxanne and Dale didn't know about our ice cream stops and unwittingly never cared to accompany us on grocery trips, but I was headed for the car as soon as I saw her clipping coupons. We treated it like it was our little secret, and I cherished those Saturdays.

There are so many other happy memories from our growing up years – of Christmas traditions and frozen-on snow boots only my mother could pry off. Our knowledge that we were adopted never seemed like anything more than a simple fact. I can't remember the first time I was told, so they must have explained it to us when we were very young. It was always the "thing" that made our family special, and they told us kids that often.

My mother met and married my father when she was eighteen and a virgin – a fact she made sure her girls knew well and heard often as we entered our teenage years. She'd recently left her childhood home in Kansas to live with her oldest sister in New York City and had gotten her first job as a line worker in a toy factory. Dad loved to tell the story about how he spotted her walking home from work one day and pulled up alongside her in his shiny red Studebaker to offer her a ride. *"And then what did she say?!"* we'd all chime together (knowing this story by heart). He'd fold his arms tightly across his chest, jut his chin up into the air and quip, *"No thank you, I'm capable of walking myself home."* And we'd laugh and laugh as though we'd never heard that story before.

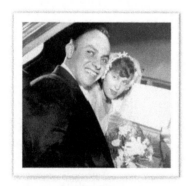
*~ His grin vs.
her hesitant look ~*

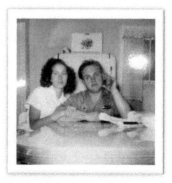
~ The young couple ~

She was the middle-ish child of nine – all girls and a boy – and an identical twin. Her father died from a heart attack in the living room of their farmhouse when she was sixteen, leaving my grandmother to raise the youngest, a toddler, by herself. Fay became second mother to my Aunt Georgia until she followed her older siblings and left home to find work and start a life of her own. Her smile was always wistful when she told us the harrowing stories of chasing after a toddler on the farm amongst the chickens, goats, and horses.

Whether it was her early indoctrination into mother-hood or it just came naturally, my mother simply loved babies. She was the one who could be counted on at church functions, social gatherings, and family outings to hold the baby – anyone's baby. Baby fussy? Hand it over to Fay. Need to round up your other two little ones? Fay'll take that baby, now you go run. We had so many photos of my mother holding someone else's baby when I was growing up that I stopped asking which one of us it was.

So once the honeymoon was over, it seemed only natural for my parents to begin building their family, and they tried for years. It wasn't that they weren't successful; they were, and regularly. Mom would get pregnant and carry the baby for a couple of months, hiding her excitement from friends and family until they felt sure they were "out of the woods." Each time they announced that they were expecting, the family would rally around them and celebrate, anticipating this most welcome addition.

But not long afterward, she'd suffer an excruciating miscarriage, leaving them deflated, heartbroken, and maybe a little ashamed. This was their painful story for a dozen years until her final pregnancy. This one looked like she was going to make it past the all-important third month and everyone started to relax, secure in the certainty of a healthy term. But then she hemorrhaged one night to a degree that frightened even my dad and they rushed her to the hospital.

I remember Dad shuddering whenever he retold the story, *"There was so much blood."* The priest was called, and they let my father stay with her overnight, since they didn't expect her to live to the next day. They didn't know until then that she'd been having ectopic pregnancies – when the fertilized egg makes its home in the Fallopian tube instead of continuing on its expected path to the uterus. As the fetus grows, the Fallopian tube can't expand enough to accommodate its increasing size and expels it in a miscarriage. Unless it bursts the tube first, which is what happened with my mother's last and final pregnancy.

She survived, and as grateful as they were, that miscarriage nearly crushed them. When I picture the 1960s version of my parents – my proud, working class father and very proper mother, humiliated because she couldn't carry a pregnancy and only ever wanted a child, I wonder at their decision to enter into the realm of adoption. Raise someone else's unwanted baby? What if the birth mother was a drug addict? Or worse? And what would the neighbors think?

But that's exactly what they did. During an era of *Leave it to Beaver* and *Please Don't Eat the Daisies,* my mom and dad forged ahead and began the process of adoption without knowing what to expect or whether their friends and family would support them.

I remember their stories about the series of interviews they endured, and how they dressed in their Sunday clothes to meet their case worker, scared to death they might say the wrong thing and be denied their chance to adopt. My dad used to laugh when he told us he had to promise to go to church with us on Sundays, which he did do, about every fifth Sunday. The other four were spent making the spaghetti sauce for dinner when we got home.

My mom and dad were close to 40 by the time they adopted me, and the joke in our family was that I'd come with the higher price tag of $157 because the cost of babies had gone up after Dale and Roxanne were each adopted. True story.

Of the three of us, I was the curious one about my background. I loved to look through my adoption papers and birth certificate and listen to them recollect how they settled on me, asking them to retell their story again and again. Apparently, my brother was of German descent and my sister was Danish. My father had been holding out for an Italian baby, and the agency called one day to tell them they had one. My hair was jet black, and Dad was ecstatic. Years later, they joked that the agency must've used shoe polish to trick them, since I grew up with reddish hair and freckles. But other than the novelty of being "chosen babies," our family acted no different than any other family I knew. My mom and dad were simply that. And my brother and sister were as much pains-in-the-asses as any of my friends' siblings.

*T*HE DEPTH OF MY DENIAL.

When I picture my mother, I see the wonderful, loving woman who raised me. The one who let me drive the four-mile straightaway to pick up my sister from soccer practice when I was still too young for my learner's permit. She made me pull over and swap seats with her before we got to the school parking lot, and I'd be grinning from ear to ear when Roxanne hopped in the back seat. And how many times had she helped me hatch a plan to talk my father into letting me have that hamster/gerbil/ mouse/fish/puppy I so desperately needed? This was the woman I saw when I referred to my mother.

And as I began navigating these tricky new waters I found myself in, I struggled between the wonderful mother in my memories and this other one whose actions I couldn't predict. Her behaviors were inconsistent and quite often offensive. She kept me off balance and uncertain. I knew I needed to step in and take control of the situation, yet I obeyed her like the child I once was, against the better judgment of the adult I'd become.

I hadn't forgotten the disciplinarian in her, and our mother/daughter dynamic hadn't changed much even though we had both aged. She was still my caring mother who in the next moment could paralyze me in her kitchen with, *"Don't you touch that,"* and block me from disinfecting her bathroom from the other side of a locked door. My 40-something self was 13 again, with braces and a training bra, being told I couldn't go to a birthday party because there'd be boys there. And therefore, I didn't.

So back to Roxanne on the phone.

34

Our new plan came together nicely, and we were feeling confident once again. Robert and I would fly from Idaho to Greenville, SC, where Roxanne would pick us up midway through her carefully timed 14-hour drive south from her apartment in western New York, and we'd all surprise Mom with a visit. Surprise!

Roxanne would then put Mom in her car and drive her back to her place "for a visit" while Robert and I would clean out her home of 20 years, pack everything up, get it ready for a realtor, and list it for sale. Figure... four or five days. Once the papers were signed, we'd drive the 3,000 miles back to Idaho, unpack her treasures into the quaint little house I'd just bought and renovated for her and arrange everything to mirror her old house, minus the clutter, fruit flies, and ants. THEN, I'd fly Roxanne and Mom out to Idaho, and together we'd ease her into her sweet new home right up the street from her loving daughter. It was a perfect plan for two siblings in total denial over what was really happening to their mother.

WELCOME TO FAY'S NEW WORLD.

The pieces fell into place pretty easily, and I was beginning to think we might actually pull this off. I found decent one-way tickets to Greenville, and Roxanne requested vacation time. Our flight was uneventful and on time, and after hanging out in airport baggage claim for half a day because she got a later start than planned and unexpected traffic, we were finally crammed into Roxanne's extremely-well-traveled SUV and heading to Canon, GA.

We hadn't seriously planned to surprise our mother, but that's precisely what happened. I'd told her we were coming. I had her write it down on her refrigerator calendar. I even confirmed that she'd written it down by having her read it back to me the night before our trip. Imagine our surprise at witnessing *her* total surprise in the driveway when she came out in her nightgown and curlers to see who had pulled in. Her first words were, *"What are you all doing here!!!??"*

I was exhausted. We'd traveled all day. Roxanne had kept us waiting in an airport for an entire afternoon. So with my newly clipped fuse, I beelined toward the kitchen to see what had gone wrong. It was right there on the calendar, "Carolyn comes," written in December. This was May. I will always regret that I snatched it off the refrigerator to point out her mistake, waggling it in front of her face to make sure she could see it. Her expression flashed between confusion and anger, and finally embarrassment, but she didn't miss a beat and snapped back that it was obviously my fault for giving her the wrong date. *Welcome to Fay's new world and brace yourself for an epic voyage, Carolyn.*

We settled in for the night on musty beds in spare bedrooms that were never prepared for guests. My poor sister had to excavate through a mountain of Holiday Barbies, still new in their unopened boxes, and mounds of saved quilting squares to unearth her bed. There was no doubt the sheets were still there from her prior year's visit when the bed had last been cleared. Robert and I got Dad's old room, which was better because at least the bed was empty, giving the appearance he had recently occupied it. Mom had clearly preserved the room exactly as he'd left it twelve years prior, sheets included. We slept on top of the covers that night.

We woke to the smell of rancid, charred something and were met by Mom's sunny greeting in her smoke-filled kitchen. Her children were home! Scorched bacon was stacked high on a coffee-stained paper plate and covered with used napkins. And very spoiled. We couldn't salvage the eggs because she was frying them in the bacon grease. We toasted bread that broke apart when we tried to remove it from the slots and reached for the peanut butter because yes, the butter on the counter had ants in it. I watched her move from toaster to coffee pot and could see the building panic on her face. Just then Robert broke the awkward silence with, *"Hey! Let's go get some breakfast! I'm buying!"*

Back from the restaurant and feeling a little more like ourselves again, the four of us crowded onto the couch in the TV room because the chairs were full of magazines and boxes. We made small talk while covertly glancing around, taking in the condition of her house in the daylight. The front living room was unusable because there was nowhere to sit there, either. Anything with a horizontal surface – couch, chairs, coffee table, end tables – was home to a stack of papers or an unopened box containing a new crockpot. I counted six of them.

No wonder Mom spent most of her time in the TV room!

But she had the blinds drawn and the only lamp on the side table didn't have a bulb in it. The TV played constant static. Mom insisted that the cable was out and that she'd been endlessly on the phone with the cable company with no resolution. She'd even *"flagged down the cable man when he drove by the house to fix it but couldn't get him to stop."* I called the 800 number and pretended to be Fay because Mom was too confused and upset to get on the line. The representative neatly informed me that "my account" hadn't been paid in five months and that I had been referred to collections.

The fire ball in my chest threatened to burst out, and I struggled to present a calm face as three sets of eyes remained fixed on me. I couldn't look at my sister or Robert because I was afraid to see my own thoughts mirrored back at me, so I casually reached for my purse and read to her my credit card number, catching my mother up on her outstanding balance.

"What are you doing?" she shrieked. *"Don't give them your credit card number! They'll steal it! And I've already sent them my money! They're a bunch of liars!"* I was becoming indoctrinated into Fay's new world at warp speed and the pit in my stomach mushroomed, steadily taking up more space until I thought I would throw it up.

In truth, I was more angry that my mother's fiscal irresponsibility had resulted in a collections referral than I was concerned that any of this was happening in the first place. My mother handled all the bills growing up, and they were paid the day they were received. My parents never even had a credit card. If you couldn't pay cash, then you didn't need it. So what in the world was going on? And why was she making such an effort to cover it with her detailed fabrications?

I slipped into her bedroom to keep myself from spewing out the venom that was building in my mouth and began quietly arranging slacks, underwear, and socks into a suitcase

I found under the bed. I needed to steel my resolve to continue on with our plan, but this "thing" that was going on with her was undermining the hope I still clung to that she was capable of some sort of independence once I got her home. Suddenly I was overcome with doubt. I felt painfully unprepared for everything being fired at me and we still hadn't figured out how we were going to get her into Roxanne's car.

With the suitcase now full, I carried it out to the side door and set it on the patio steps for Roxanne to sneak into her trunk. I spotted Mom's purse hanging on a doorknob and reached for it to add it to her things. It was unnaturally light when I lifted it, like it was a spare from another season, so I snapped it open to look inside. My mind raced as I dug through the cavernous, empty space, trying to make sense of it. No wallet, no coins, just wadded up Kleenex and some Good Housekeeping subscription renewal cards occupied the darkness.

Our travel plans to Idaho had just come to a grinding halt as I realized there was no ID in her purse to board a plane. With no strategy in my head and a body coiled in dread, I left the bedroom and headed straight for the TV room, purse swinging from my wrist.

Another thing I regret, looking back, is how I carried it out to her and asked if it was hers. *"Of course it's mine,"* she said, reaching out to snatch it away. I plunked it down in front of her, *"Then where's your wallet, Mom? Your driver's license? Your money?"* Grabbing the purse, she dug into it and came up looking so confused that I was instantly sorry for my accusatory tone. She hurtled herself into the front living room and began tearing into her credenza, stuffed full to the top with unopened mail and clipped newspaper articles. She moved on to her dresser drawers, kitchen drawers, everything, searching for the lost items.

Emotions escalated within minutes, with her insisting

someone had been in her house and stolen everything from her purse. Regret #36, I volleyed right back and challenged, *"So this intruder apparently didn't want anything else in your house, right? Like your car keys or any of your valuables? They just sat down, rummaged through your purse, and then left?"*

Imagine that everything your loved one says to you is delivered with sincere conviction. They're definitely not imagining things – they'll tell you that. And they're absolutely certain that what they see, hear, and feel are true.

Do you think maybe you would pause and consider that you might be making a huge mistake by uprooting them from their home? Would you doubt your own judgment and worry that perhaps things aren't as bad as they appear – that maybe it's *you* who's overreacting and might even be making things worse? That if you give them a little more leeway to make a few more concrete mistakes, maybe then you'll be convinced it's time to take action?

There are things we look back on and wish we had done differently. I wish I had been given more time to prepare for this. I wish I would've known how to recognize the signs and been shown how to appropriately and lovingly respond to the madness as it surrounded me *before* it began to engulf me. And even as I say this, I can imagine someone rolling their eyes and scoffing, convinced they would've caught on sooner and been more decisive in arriving at their own plan of action. But these were very new shoes I was walking in, and likely as uncomfortable a fit for an outside observer, I think.

On the other hand, you may have witnessed enough to deem your loved one unable to live alone and confidently start planning what to do next. That's a reassuring emotional place to start, for sure. You can at least move forward with conviction, secure in your decision. But when it came to my mother, things came at me a little at a time and at different speeds. Like waves on the beach, one new and strange behavior rolled in right after the last, never really crashing, but relentless. Just when I thought the water was calming, another wave washed onto the shore, always a little worse than the last, followed by yet another. But I was so focused on signs of smoother water the previous waves didn't register in my brain as alarming enough to warrant decisive action.

She was like a grease fire in your kitchen. You manage to snuff it out, only to find your sleeve is on fire, and as you plunge your arm into the sink full of water, the flames explode to the curtains above it. Each new fire she lit, once blotted out, would rekindle and spread in another direction. And right after I doused the last one, I would tell myself this had to be it, that there couldn't possibly be another behind it. But even when I was blessed with a short reprieve, one would mysteriously reignite.

I was so focused on each little catastrophe that I didn't completely absorb the severity of her situation. I compartmentalized each one and dealt with it singularly. By not looking at them as a whole, I never had that "Aha!" moment of "Mom needs more help than I'm able to give."

At least not then, I didn't. Her new behaviors were so troubling that I remained off balance and doubted every decision I made (or didn't make) about her care. And this move to Idaho was already beginning to feel like a huge mistake that I couldn't undo.

It took a metaphoric towering inferno to move me to action, something that still leaves me in awe when I play back these stories of just what it was like for me in the beginning.

Maybe my hesitancy to fully assess my mother's situation could be better described as a "lack of ability" to fully assess. How *could* I know? I was certainly no professional. I'd had no training in the world of dementia. I could blame myself, and without a doubt I did, but as I listen to the same revelations now from conversations I have with people who are experiencing the beginnings of dementia with their own loved ones,

I've come to realize that this disease is more than just incredibly cruel, it's gradual and it's very sneaky.

Those people with their wide-eyed expressions and predictably shocked tones of voice are all so familiar to me now. I nod my head and listen sympathetically as they recount their own stories as though no one could ever imagine their last horror. *"That happened to you, too?!"* they'd ask, *"I can't believe I said that to them! I feel like the worst son/daughter/ wife/husband for responding that way. I'm a terrible person."*

S UBTERFUGE AND A ROLL OFF DUMPSTER.

It was time to implement the next part of our plan – Roxanne and Fay's long drive to New York. Robert and I needed her out of the house so we could get busy clearing it out. The morning after discovering she had no ID, no money, and no insurance card, we ushered her into the car with her suitcase hidden in the trunk and a purse full of Kleenex. We smiled and waved goodbye as they pulled out of the driveway, both of us taking a collective breath as we watched her bobbing head and confused smile disappear down the road. It was too late now for her to refuse to go. We simply packed her up and hustled her out.

None of us could begin to know how this was going to shake out, but it seemed like the only way to proceed for us to continue moving forward. We had work to do, and we could already tell it wasn't going to be a four- or five-day job like we'd thought. With Mom out of the way, the first thing I did was call the local U-Haul office.

After answering a few questions about Mom's possessions and the size of her house, I reserved their 26-foot truck, good for a complete household with three bedrooms. Then I ordered a 12-yard roll-off dumpster to be placed in the driveway for all the items that didn't make the cut for the move and couldn't be donated. This thing was huge. You could walk straight into it from one end and keep walking in great strides before you got to the other end. We knew it was overkill, but we didn't want to be slowed down by having to reorder another dumpster midway through our clean out.

That roll-off dumpster had to be removed and replaced three times.

The guy at the U-Haul garage proved to be a lifesaver, considering the monumental bad start we had together. He and Robert butted heads within the first five minutes in his front office. Bubba's (no, I'm not making this up) Southern accent was so thick that Robert couldn't understand him and kept repeating, *"What?"* but in a way that clearly implied he was from the great Northwest and quite separate from Bubba's deep South. He said it enough times that finally Bubba turned his reddened face to me, spat into his Styrofoam cup, and said he'd just realized he didn't have a truck for me after all.

Actual walls felt like they were caving in on me and my chest was collapsing along with it. I inhaled what breath I could and asked Bubba to come with me outside. I pointed as we walked along the trucks, *"What about this one? Or this one? I'm really in a jam here. We're moving my mom out of her house, and it's packed with a lifetime of stuff. We can't take it all with us. Do you know anyone who would be interested in the things we don't take? Furniture, everything, they can have it for free..."*

And after a half-dozen signatures and the swipe of my credit card, I followed Robert out of the U-Haul yard; he in our brand new 26-foot truck that would carry us across the United States, and I in my mom's car with the front right tire thub-thubbing, the result of some unknown contact she'd made with something that apparently didn't budge when she hit it. Behind ME was Bubba in his spare 26-foot U-Haul truck designated for all the items that weren't coming with us and his buddy following at the rear to give him a ride back to the garage.

By the afternoon of Day Two and the second roll-off

dumpster, half of our U-Haul was filled and Bubba's U-Haul was completely packed. Bubba showed up within 30 minutes of my call, looked inside his truck, our truck, the house, and said, *"You're gonna need more help."*

The next morning, Bubba and his huge brother-in-law, Tiny (pronounced Tah'Nee), replaced his full U-Haul with another 26-footer and an old pickup truck. By lunchtime, two men from Bubba's garage showed up to help us load them. I think we both could have cried.

We ordered a pizza for lunch, and I ran to the gas station for a case of beer – anything to keep them there and happy. It was a full afternoon of, *"Watcha gone do wit dis piece? Dat piece? You gone keep dat?"* I became director and choreographer, pointing to which truck each item went, making ten second decisions and intentionally relaxing my shoulders as I watched childhood memories get packed into a truck I'd never see again. My heart was sick for my mother, but our own truck was almost full, and we still had more rooms to clear out.

It was sometime near the end of Day Three when they found the freezers. Four of them, not counting the kitchen refrigerator/freezer. They were on the back screened porch, humming along, packed solid, like ice pick solid. You'd think they'd found pirate chests – buried treasure. I told them all four were going into the roll-off unless they wanted them, and that I couldn't vouch for the food inside. Turned out they were going to keep the meat for their dogs and sell the freezers. Enterprising capitalists, they were, and more power to them.

Their first order of business was to dolly them out to the yard and prop open the doors. It took a full day in the sun for things to thaw enough to chip into and look around. We found an entire ring of keys and a sixteen-year-old ham among other strange and intriguing things in those chests, like bags of frozen corn with dates on them that could only mean my parents had hauled them with them during their move from New York in 1992. This was 2012. Of all the riches that went into Bubba's U-Hauls, the freezers were by far the true gems for these guys, and it was fun to watch them unearth each new nugget and deliberate over its mysterious history.

Sometime during Day Four, a man showed up at the side door and said he'd heard we were hauling things out and could he take a look in my father's workshop. We'd already scoured through it and saved a few things, but Dad, like Mom, had been a master collector. He kept inches of cut copper pipe, *"You never know when you're going to need a small piece,"* and stacked blocks of wood in various sizes on shelves labeled by their dimensions. He had every kind of hand tool dating back to the Great Depression when his father was a stone smith. He'd even kept the lead wool no longer used for old cast iron pipe joints from his young plumbing days in a wooden box under his workbench. Ten minutes later, our visitor was back at the side door, *"I'll clean that entire workshop out for you and even sweep if I can haul it all away."* Square deal, and with both parties feeling like we'd won the lottery, we shook hands.

Things were slowing down by Day Five or Six and we were getting down to the real junk and our third roll-off. We could sense that Bubba's guys were losing their enthusiasm and we were about to be back on our own with this mess.

They pulled out of the driveway that evening, everyone waving goodbye and shouting, *"Thank you!!"* for all our separate reasons. We'd just spent two or three complete days with them, eating all our meals together and joking around while we worked, and as we watched them disappear down the road, it felt like the wind in our sails went with them. They'd never met my mother, but before they were through, they knew her well enough to laugh at all her collections and kid about how many cans of cream of mushroom soup one woman could cram into her pantry.

Day Seven and it was just the two of us again. The third roll-off was back in primary use and we'd begun simply pitching things over the side instead of wasting time carrying items in from one end. Seriously, McCormick spices from 1984? You couldn't even smell the cinnamon in the square tin anymore. Jams and canned vegetables that were easily 25 years old and clearly carted there from New York. Runny face cream, toothpaste hardened solid in the tube, Listerine bottles with globular clouds bobbing around inside. Even the Q-tips looked dirty in their container. We found an unopened box of Ritz Crackers shoved up inside Mom's bathroom vanity with puckered print and mold on the cardboard from getting repeatedly dripped on from a leak that had never been fixed.

There was a case of shrimp flavored ramen noodles under her bed, along with Dad's shaving kit, suspenders, and a bottle of cologne. Once we mined through the debris stacked on top of the washer and dryer, we discovered bags of store brand potato chips with red 99-cent clearance stickers on them stuffed inside both drums. I counted 19 bags. The smell of rancid oil assaulted our noses as we opened the lid to the washing machine. It must've leeched through the unopened cellophane bags and leaked into the drums. What struck me most wasn't that she'd been hoarding 19 bags of chips in her washer and dryer, but realizing that she couldn't have been doing laundry since the time those bags had been stuffed inside.

And the beans – old milk gallons and plastic tubs and sticky twist-tie bags full of every shape, size, and color of dried beans. The tubs were so old the lids crackled into pieces when we lifted them to look inside. We couldn't in good conscience donate any of this, so it all got tossed into the roll-off.

It was finally time to tackle Mom's closet. The metal accordion doors were jammed so tightly shut from whatever was packed behind them that we had to remove them from their hinges. Inside was a solid wall of clothes. Jeans were on hangers and so crowded that you couldn't remove one hanger without disrupting the entire section. Money was stuffed into the pockets randomly. Not a lot, but tens and twenties spread out just enough to tempt us into shoving our hands into them before we moved them to the box for the church. I lost count of the dresses with tags still on them, yet her shoes looked like they were from another period – outdated, heels scrubbed bare, their leather cracked. I sat down on the floor among them, fingering the worn areas her bunions had made as I puzzled over my Depression-era mother, frugality her entire way of life, buying dresses she never wore while deciding she didn't need or deserve a new pair of shoes.

My mind traveled back to my school years and her old blue winter coat. That thing came out of the closet every October of my youth. The first thing I bought her after I'd landed a real job out of college was a puffy new stadium jacket (Christmas, 1987). I remember my pride at presenting to her this new, stylish coat with my hard-earned money. Her response? *"It's nice, but I wish you wouldn't have wasted your money. There's nothing wrong with my blue coat."*

With the jeans and dresses now cleared out, the wooden hanging bar looked grotesquely naked and sagged like it had been slapped down by life. A stack of vintage Samsonite luggage was piled high at the back of her closet, and I wondered out loud where exactly my mother had planned to travel these past twenty years. As I excavated through the pile, one of the cases felt unusually weighty and off balance as I maneuvered it out to the front. Maybe this was where she hid the silver! So far, we'd found nothing of value in the house, and hope sparked a tiny flicker in my heart, since the cost of Mom's move had fallen onto my shoulders, and my stack of receipts was about to require a bigger rubber band.

The metal latch unsnapped with a sharp click, and I laid

open the case on the floor, revealing a black plastic box about half the size of a shoebox (and heavy!).

I was already wrangling the lid off when I saw the letters "SAL" scratched into one side with something sharp. I let out a shriek as I dropped the box to the floor and shot backwards out of the closet, crab-crawling to the far wall. It sat there between me and the door, that ominous black cube, sure to spring open on its own any second.

My scream brought Robert bounding into the bedroom, ready to battle whatever it was I'd just uncovered. He stopped short when he spotted the box and then me, pressed up against the wall, and started to laugh. Bending, he snatched up the box and turned it over to read the letters on the side, *"Poor Sal, you've been relegated to the closet for what, twelve years?"* And after only a minute of consideration, it was decided that Dad would take his place of honor up front with us on the ride back home. It was the least we could do for him.

With Mom's bedroom finally quarried, I felt ready for a new challenge. We'd finally exposed some surfaces in the kitchen, so I began to clean. Not the spray Windex kind of clean – more like the tie-a-bandanna-over-your-face-and-strap-on-some-gloves-while-using-one-of-Dad's-putty-knives-and-bleach kind of clean.

We'd rescheduled our real estate agent's appointment twice already because the house was still a shameful wreck. Then one evening she dropped by unannounced, *"Just to see how y'all are doing,"* and perhaps to make sure we hadn't changed our minds about listing with her.

She was sweet, gracious, and very southern. Her arms remained folded across her chest as I showed her around the house. Her polite smile never faltered, but it couldn't conceal her look of unease and maybe even a little revulsion while I explained that I was sure we could clear out the rest of the rubbish and get rid of that strange smell before she came back to put up her sign. We just needed a few more days. I hated seeing my parents' home through her eyes. Her expression reflected back to me a house that had deteriorated from a place of pride to a sad and neglected bit of a shit box.

This depressing little house had once been their source of happiness, from Dad's workshop to Mom's garden. It was exactly right for them. At $55,000, they couldn't believe their luck that they could afford to pay cash for it from the sale of our family home in New York, and it only needed a few things. Dad was handy and still able to do most of the work himself. After hardwood floors, new kitchen appliances (now two decades old), and new carpet in the TV room (also two decades old now and maybe a little peed on), they settled into their new home and anticipated living out their golden years.

Our sweet, frozen-faced Realtor suggested we list for $49,000, but that we shouldn't expect anywhere near full price. Assuming, of course, we could actually produce a clean, empty house for her as promised.

Meanwhile, we had been receiving our morning and evening *"What is taking you so long!?"* calls from my sister. Bless her heart, she'd been going through her own trials with our mom. Their long drive north had turned into an endless interrogation, with Fay holding the spotlight over her captive driver. Roxanne was so exhausted from fielding the constant stream of questions that she knew she couldn't make it home without stopping. She took a chance and called our cousin in Virginia, Ruth Ann, and said hello after 30-odd years of not saying hello.

Cousin Ruth Ann was more than just happy to hear from them. She was ecstatic to have Roxanne and Fay stop for the night to see her mother (Mom's sister), Darlene. Since they were going to be passing through midway home, Roxanne hoped that a brief visit between the two sisters who hadn't seen each other in years might distract Fay enough to give her a break for a night.

That was probably the best move my sister made. I can only imagine now how incredibly alone she must've felt, trapped in the car with our now-raging mother and dodging scary questions she didn't know how to answer. The support and warmth of a welcoming family unit was her bit of respite on an impossibly long trip and likely gave her the resolve to complete it. For our mother, it would be the last time she would see her sister, though none of us knew it then.

I never really had "the extended family experience" growing up. You would think that with five living aunts, each with plenty of kids around our age, we would've always been surrounded by relatives, but our family was geographically scattered just enough to keep us from doing much visiting or ever really getting to know each other as a clan. Cell phones with unlimited data plans hadn't been invented, and social media was a term no one had heard of yet. My father received only one week's vacation each year, so Mom's sisters remained low on his priority list and would maybe be fit into some weekend road trip.

As a teenager, I remember feeling like the odd-man-out whenever my friends talked about huge family holidays or hanging out with their cousins. So as an adult, I was always surprised and felt a little awkward when I received a Facebook friend request from some random relative I hadn't seen since I was maybe 11 or 12. Some I'd never met. They'd write to me with such enthusiasm and inquire about my mother, sharing stories from memories they had from one of our summer visits when they were a kid. They might not have seen her in over three decades, but their messages were always heartfelt and loving.

By the time Mom and Roxanne arrived in Virginia, Ruth Ann had managed to gather up Aunt Darlene, Aunt Georgia (who'd been visiting from Oregon), and their collective families to await Mom's arrival. Within minutes of sitting down at the kitchen table filled with photo albums, cookies, and a pot of coffee, my mother glanced from one sister to the other and said, *"I don't know any of you. You're all so gray."*

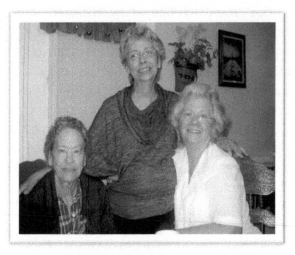

~ L to R: Fay, Aunt Georgia, Aunt Darlene ~

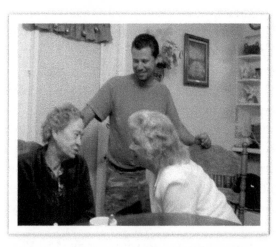

~ L to R: Fay, cousin Gabriel, Aunt Darlene ~

Notice Fay, also-gray, sitting in the group. They all just laughed and continued catching up until Mom nodded off at the table and they put her to bed. Roxanne and Fay left in the morning after coffee and toast, with everyone promising to keep in better touch from then on.

They reached New York after midnight and settled into my sister's two-bedroom apartment, now very full with our mother, Roxanne's daughter, son-in-law, and their four young children. Mom was given the second bedroom so she'd be more comfortable while everyone else spread out on couches and the floor, camping style. My sister had already taken as much vacation time as the post office would allow, so she had no choice but to return to work the next day. Leaving Mom with her daughter and the kids seemed like an easy enough task for just eight hours, so she set her alarm and crept out in the dark the next morning while everyone still slept.

Sometime during the day, though, Mom disappeared. She wasn't missed until my sister got home and asked where Grandma was. Her daughter thought she was lying down in Roxanne's room, and we never did figure out how long she'd been gone. When my sister called 911 to report an elderly woman missing, the dispatcher told her they already had my mother in a holding location and were waiting for the incoming call. The police had found her in the Wegman's parking lot, wandering between the cars and jiggling door handles. She was waiting for Roxanne in a conference room at the sheriff's office, sitting erect in her chair and indignant over being manhandled in a grocery store parking lot when all she was doing was looking for her car.

A safeguard was put into place the next day. A friend of my sister's agreed to Fay-sit for the day until she got home. Everything seemed okay until Mom asked the friend why she was hanging around all day and the friend, unschooled in the value of a well-crafted fib, told her exactly why she was there. Mom stood up after hearing she'd been assigned a babysitter, let herself into the bathroom and locked the door. She stayed in there (the only bathroom in the apartment), refusing to open the door until Roxanne came home that evening and convinced her to come out.

None of us had figured out yet how easy (and preferable) it was to lie to a person with dementia.

*D*EMENTIA – *WE HADN'T EVEN BEGUN USING THAT WORD YET.*

During those early days we honestly thought our mother was just being difficult. A cranky little spitfire and a general pain in the butt. Those were the signs of getting "senile," which we'd always interchanged with "old." Neither my sister nor I had any experience dealing with someone with dementia, so neither of us could've predicted how the future was going to look. We didn't have a clue what to expect. We were busy with what was being thrown at us today, and that was how we lived every day in the beginning.

Sometime during her stay at the apartment, a disaster occurred that nearly unraveled every plan we'd made to relocate Mom to Idaho. I'd managed to unearth a photocopy of her birth certificate, a portion of her expired Georgia driver's license with the corner cut off (thank God Mom saved everything – *did I just say that?*), and a copy of her application for a replacement Social Security card, minus the card. It wasn't the required airport ID to secure our mother a flight, but it was all we had, and it was worth gold to us. I'd already called airport security from my mother's house in Georgia and explained our situation. All they would say was, *"Arrive at Security early with the documents and hope for the best."*

I FedExed everything in an envelope to Roxanne, which she proceeded to hide under her mattress. Apparently that was the choicest, least obvious place to hide something as incredibly important and integral to the successful passage of my mother from New York to Idaho as these documents were.

And the next day the envelope was gone. Evidently my sister's most-excellent hiding spot was an equally favored looking spot of Fay's.

She called me with the news on something like Day Seven or Eight. I remember we'd been sweating for days because the A/C had died and grime clung to us as we dug out closets and cabinets, adding to our sour moods. I answered my phone, ready for another litany of questions as to why we were taking so long. I *wasn't* expecting this. *"Roxanne! That was everything we had! And we don't even know if it was going to be enough!"* She was crying. I swallowed my next words and instead told her I was sure she'd find the envelope and to keep looking. She said she'd looked everywhere already but would start over. We ended the call on a note of uncertainty and anguish so heavy it was difficult to breathe.

Two more days of panicked searching and Roxanne uncovered the envelope from the bottom of the bathroom cabinet, under bottles of peroxide, toilet cleaner, and tampons – Mom's likewise careful choice for safe-keeping. We decided Roxanne would move the envelope to the trunk of her car, where only she had the key.

Emotions seemed to settle in the apartment over the next several days and things returned to a predictable pace. Mom became more involved with the girls as she was reintroduced to her "new grandkids." I remember one afternoon Roxanne called me on speaker phone to tell me Mom was making pancakes for the whole crew. I could hear squeals of laughter from all four grandkids and my heart melted for my mother. She was doing her favorite things again – cooking for a crowd and being surrounded by children.

We could finally see progress being made at Mom and Dad's house. Carpets were scheduled for cleaning, lawn service was arranged, and I was making headway on all the sticky surfaces. We were beginning to feel like we were finally on the other side of this mountain we'd been climbing.

Every time I uncovered some overdue invoice, I'd call the number, inquire how far behind "I was," settle up, and then cancel. I learned that Fay was a platinum member of the Policemen's Giving Campaign and officer Jake was going to be *"very sad to lose you as a loyal supporter."* She was an auto renewal subscriber to Publisher's Clearing House Seed Catalog. *Publisher's Clearing House has a seed catalog?!* How many "World's Most Amazing Brownies" cookbooks does one person need? Fay needed seven, apparently, at $39.99 each, and she was receiving collection notices.

Mail was forwarded, the cable was canceled, and the neighbors were notified, each promising to keep an eye on the house. It was Day Eleven.

With the last bag of trash thrown into the very full dumpster and the living room lights turned on so it looked like someone was home, I mopped my way from the back of the house straight out the front door. We threw the key under the mat and launched the dirty mop over the side of the roll-off before climbing into our tightly packed U-Haul, Dad riding shotgun under the passenger seat.

We were exhausted, aching, and hungry. There'd been nothing in the house to eat since the first day we began moving Mom's things and witnessed just how atrocious her living conditions were. We'd tossed everything, bleached everything, and had nothing to store food in – the poor kitchen refrigerator never cooled again after we'd cleaned it. It had been leaking brown ooze and smelled so bad when we first arrived that we hauled it out into the yard to be emptied and disinfected first thing. It simply gave out after that (we joked that we'd killed it with kindness).

We'd been living on Subway sandwiches because they were the only meals we could get fast, were consistently good, and offered up some variety of vegetables. We hadn't cooked anything. How could we? We couldn't bring ourselves to eat off any of the dishes. It felt like the entire house was contaminated.

It's hard to describe the unsettling feeling of attempting to drink from a cup that smells like sour milk as you raise it to your mouth, or of grabbing a bowl from the cupboard that sticks to the one beneath it. We couldn't convince ourselves to drink the water from the tap that seemed to sputter and hiss when the handle was turned, so we bought bottled water instead. We were constantly buying ice for the new Styrofoam cooler I bought at the Shop-N-Save to keep the bottles cold. We didn't even consider using one of the half-dozen plastic coolers we found in the garage for all the reasons you can imagine by now. It was like we were surrounded by stale, spoiling awfulness, and we couldn't scrub it off or shower it away.

Who could blame me for fantasizing about food by then? It didn't even have to be fancy – the thought of any food could hold my attention for hours. I commenced regaling Robert with stories about Waffle House, the most ubiquitous restaurant in the South, next to Cracker Barrel I suppose. I couldn't wait to introduce him to it, with their line cooks standing just feet away from you as they cracked countless eggs into butter filled skillets, the edges crisping over open flames. You could smell cinnamon raisin toast and fresh coffee when you walked through the door as they greeted you with, *"Hey Sugar, take any seat."* I could recite almost anything on the menu, and those syrupy salty pancakes! I craved their hot grits with a melting pat of butter floating on top and thin, crispy bacon you could pick up with your fingers and snap off between your teeth. It became our recurring conversation during the last of our worst days in that house, and something we both looked forward to. More than anything, I wanted Robert to experience the famous "Scattered, Smothered, and

Covered." San Diego Boy had never been there, and the fact that we were going to pass right by one at the highway entrance filled me with excitement and anticipation.

Just a few miles after pulling out of Mom's driveway we approached the highway on-ramp with the entrance to the Waffle House on the right. Robert slowed the truck, blinkers flashing, and came to a stop at the entrance. He didn't make the turn in, deeming it too tight for the 26-foot truck to maneuver. I was sure there was plenty of room, but he didn't think so and was annoyed that I pushed him to try, saying I cared more about a Waffle House than the difficulty it was going to be for him to get us there.

And just like that we both exploded into a back-and-forth volley of accusations, blocking any unsuspecting breakfast seekers from entering the parking lot and getting their hot cup of coffee and pancakes. We just sat there, both of us seething, with him feeling like I was being incredibly selfish and me feeling utterly misunderstood. How could this scenario have gone any other way, really? We'd been holding it together for days and collapsing into bed at night, only to do it all over again the next day under the filthiest conditions. All I wanted was to treat him to something I knew he'd enjoy. It was my way of showing him how appreciated he was. All he wanted was to successfully complete his job and get us safely on the road, and possibly as far and as fast from that house as he could.

They say hindsight is easy. The sad part is that it comes afterward and is usually accompanied by regret. My regret is that my eyes only saw that I could do nothing right. That even the smallest gesture of thanks from me was going to be rebuffed by Robert in some covert effort of his to show me just how inconvenienced and put upon he was during this whole undertaking. My guilt over my mother's monumental mess was so overpowering that I held sentry over him, constantly searching for any hint of revealing itself in Robert's actions. A therapist would call that a classic anger-guilt split (yes, I looked it up, and it's referenced in the back of the book).

"She's not going to be any better in the new house."

We settled into our routine somehow, and by our second or third day on the road, and after rehashing every disturbing detail, Robert broached the topic of what to do with Fay once she arrived in Idaho. *"What do you mean, 'What do we do with her?' We set her up in her house and I check in on her. Like we planned! Right?"* I couldn't hide my panic.

"Sweetheart, your mom is worse than either of us thought. I don't think you're really looking at the true picture. She's not going to be any better in the new house than she was in Georgia," he said.

And... Three. Two. One. I could feel the hot flush wash entirely over me. Complete. Utter. Meltdown. How could he just announce this as we're heading toward our destination, our plan only halfway completed? It had been in motion for weeks, and now he's claiming it won't work? And what the HELL are we supposed to do as an alternative?! My mother is crammed into a two-bedroom apartment in New York with three other adults and four children. My sister is waiting for the signal to remove her swiftly to Idaho. I bought a house, for Pete's sake. We spent months renovating it for her. How exactly does Plan B fit into all this? We don't even have a Plan B! My mind reeled. He was being so negative! He didn't understand! He didn't support me! Why was he being such an *asshole*!?

A torrent of emotions raged through me like a forest fire, burning anywhere my veins fed. My heart hammered in my chest, and my lungs felt too full to draw a decent breath. Were we really going to fight again?

All I wanted was his support, and to me that meant sticking to our plan. Anything else felt like treason. I had just witnessed conditions I never imagined I'd link with my mother, and my head wasn't in a good place to brainstorm another way to fix this. We'd been through this a hundred times already and *there were no other strategies to consider.* We were implementing the only option we could find available. You can say I had blinders on, but it was simply all I could do to stay afloat by keeping our plan in play. I think I was shell shocked from everything I'd had to do those past weeks just to be in this truck heading west. And we hadn't even gotten to the hard part.

"But hadn't Robert dropped everything to fly across the United States with you, Carolyn? Didn't he just spend eleven days immersed in filth and decay, working tirelessly until he collapsed into bed every night?

Apparently I *had* forgotten all of that. The only way I seemed able to view our current situation was from the darkness of my wounded emotional corner, so that's what I did. I clung hard to my hurt feelings, nursing my righteous indignation and not giving much consideration to how Robert must be feeling. I think we spent the entire drive across Wyoming in silence. Wyoming is a really wide state.

Our drive dragged on for days, with each one pretty much the same as the last. We'd drive until dusk, look for hotels online and book one with easy access that looked closest to the highway. Then we'd survey the parking lot to find the best way to park the behemoth 26-footer so that it wouldn't block people and wasn't at risk for theft. This was our evening ritual. Pull forward, back up, pull forward some more and finally settle into a space under a security light or backed up to a dumpster so the rear door couldn't be jimmied open.

Then we'd order something mediocre from the hotel menu, shower, set the alarm for 6am, and pass out.

We pulled into town on Day Six of our drive, and all I wanted to do was put it in park and get out. All Robert wanted to do was drive down the hill to the feed store and put the truck on the grain scales. *"Are you joking? I don't care how much it weighs! I just want to get OUT."* What I really wanted was to get into bed and stay there for three days. So of course we drove down the hill to the feed store and put the truck on the scales.

I did learn a few things while we were there. Our truck was rated for 26,000 lbs., and we were over that by 600. This was more than just an interesting tidbit that I assumed he was only curious about. *"You realize we just drove 3,000 miles through 8 states illegally overweight, right?"* he asked. *"An accident wouldn't have been covered by our insurance, we would've been liable for any damage to our truck, their vehicle, or we could've just killed someone."* Robert admitted he'd been worrying about it for six days and didn't want to tell me. There was nothing we could've done about it, but now that it was over, he just had to know, and he'd guessed right.

We chugged back up the hill to my mother's new house, lowered the truck ramp, and it started to rain. My best friend Rhonda was waiting for us as we pulled up. She took one look at the solid wall of possessions stacked to the ceiling behind the truck door and said, *"We need more people."* Our friends Jeff and Ginny showed up with rain slickers on within an hour of my panicked message left on their voicemail. The five of us trudged up and down the slippery wet ramp as the rain grew steadier with as many boxes and other items as each could carry. We're talking about a packed-to-the-gills 26-foot moving truck. Have I mentioned that already? We could've used five *more* people, but I was hesitant to make those calls. (Yes, I am my mother's daughter, and well trained to not ask for help.)

We needed to hurry. I'd purchased the airline tickets for my mother and sister a week earlier and had underestimated the time needed to drive back and then prepare for them. They were arriving in the morning, and we still had to empty the truck, unpack boxes, assemble beds, and set up the kitchen. And it was getting dark.

My phone had been vibrating in my pocket but my hands were full each time, so I stacked a new box in the living room, forgot about it, and returned to the truck. I felt it buzz again and this time stopped to check the screen. It was my sister. They'd landed at their connection in Phoenix, and something was terribly wrong. Her words came fast and became steadily shriller as she stammered through her description of the first leg of their trip.

"Roxanne, slow down. What's going on?"

- She won't get on the plane.

"What do you mean? Just tell her she's coming to see me for a visit and she's halfway there," I said.

- I tried that! She says she knows what I'm up to and she's not having any of it. She locked herself in a bathroom stall and won't come out.

That was Roxanne's reality. My reality was that I'd just answered her call in the rain with a box on one hip while smashing the phone between my cheek and shoulder to keep it from dropping onto the driveway. It was pouring now, and I was holding up the moving line as I watched water get all over my mother's newly sanded-and-polyurethaned living room floor. We'd just driven across the United States for six days after spending two weeks in Hell at Mom's and I was having trouble mustering up enough fucks for her.

"Well, I guess she's yours then."

- (Silence.)

"If you can't get her here, you'll just have to take her back home with you," I said.

- (Crickets.)

Her text arrived early the next morning saying they'd landed just as I entered the traffic pattern for airport arrivals and departures.

I'd left the house before dawn for the two-hour drive to the airport, leaving Ginny, another friend Kim, and her mother Betty still unpacking dishes and making beds. They had roughly five hours to get everything in order before we walked through the front door, and it didn't look like they were going to make it.

"WHERE ARE YOU TAKING ME AGAIN?"

They were standing at the curb as I pulled up. Mom looked like a frazzled little chicken, and Roxanne looked like she could cry. Everyone was exhausted. They'd both flown all night, I'd just unpacked and set up an entire house's contents, and Mom was beyond confused. The entire drive home from the airport was filled with, *"Where are we going again?" "Where are you taking me again?" "Are we there yet?" "How much longer?"* To every parent who has suffered a road trip to the Grand Canyon, Niagara Falls, or over the river and through the woods to Grandmother's house – I get it now. I ran out of cheery answers after question number 27 and began calculating the ramifications of pulling over and shaking the next one out of her. After 110 miles and three bathroom stops, each one a precious guess as to whether she'd get back in the car, we finally pulled up to the front of Fay's new home and everyone hobbled out onto the sidewalk.

We entered through the front door to a tidier, cleaner version of her home in Georgia. The boxes that never got unpacked were stowed away in the basement, stacked in neat rows in a far corner behind a locked door that made it off limits to my mother. The house looked perfect.

I quietly guided her through her new home and held my breath, carefully scanning her face for any sign of a scowl, twitch, or alarm. Her bedrooms looked lovely with her quilts on the beds and her bedside lamps turned on. Her old mantle clock ticked steadily over the fireplace.

Her living room couch fit perfectly with her favorite coffee table and chair, and the kitchen looked like it was meant to hold her enameled kitchen table and chairs, with coffee cups hanging on a vintage rack we'd found packed away in her old pantry that had made the cut and into our 26-footer. Neither of us said a word throughout the tour until I finally broke the silence with a half-whispered, *"Well, what do you think, Mom?"*

She glanced around the room one more time before turning to me with, *"How did these people get all of my things?"*

How does one explain to their mother that they'd just emptied her house of all her possessions, moved the choicest items cross country, chucked the rest, and moved her into a strange house far away from everything and everyone she knows because we think she's losing her mind?

You lie to her like it's a solid fact, plain and simple. The problem was I didn't understand that tidbit yet, and I certainly hadn't learned how to actually do it.

Resources *were* available, including books about dealing with diseases of the aging brain – I just hadn't read any of them up until then. I was too busy being indoctrinated by fire into the world of dementia and was otherwise occupied, combating one volcanic mess after another while planning my next move. My head was down, and I was grinding forward, taking not one minute to stop and consider that I needed the help of some experts. I felt like I was batting back tennis balls from some misfiring machine stuck in the fast mode.

Each new situation I experienced with her came as a surprise to me, and it often required a response without hesitation, or I'd be caught in a lie, and believe me, she was watching. This was foreign territory – *how could I look her in the eyes and lie to this woman who raised me not to lie,* without her catching me, and with who-knows-what kind of penalty to pay if I did get caught?

So I responded with simply, *"Isn't it lovely?"*

Over time I discovered the power of our local library, chock full of resource books on dementia. I began showing up every few days in search of new books that might help me figure out what to do with this stranger inside my mother's body. I would've sat right down on the floor there and devoured each one if I'd had the time, but my days had morphed into something akin to balancing the demands of two lives wrapped into one. My only opportunity to read was right before I passed out in bed each night.

Some of the books were helpful, but most missed the mark for me. I was looking for real life stories from adult children who had discovered their parent in the early, most frightening stages of dementia, and what they did next. Who could guide me through the quagmire of accusations, distrust, and confusion? That's what I was searching for on those crammed shelves in the non-fiction section.

I got lucky here and there, with some books providing bits of advice that I connected with. *"Don't argue the facts with them – it only causes confusion and aggravation."* And *"Don't excite them with raised voices and rapid movements."* And *"If things start to escalate and tempers flare, do your best to distract them with another, more pleasant subject or try a question on some topic with which they're well-versed."* I clung to those recommendations, but I longed to hear the actual scenarios behind each one. Had these people been going through similar situations as I was now? Were they crying every day? Did they constantly doubt themselves? I needed real stories!

The 36-Hour Day by Nancy L. Mace, MA and Peter V. Rabins, MD, MPH came closest to helping me, but it seemed to give examples of more advanced dementia behaviors than what my mother was exhibiting. I still needed more practical help with the heated accusations, meanness, and especially how to lie to her with a straight face.

To: Carolyn
From: Rhonda

How are things going? Has your mom figured out how to get down to the basement yet? It just seems like a matter of time. My friend owns an Alzheimer's assisted living home in Reno, and she posted this on FB. It's kind of what we were talking about the other day.
Source: Alzheimer's Association

Caregiver/Person with dementia Interaction Tips
• Use simple and exact words
• Reassure, reassure, reassure
• Do not disagree or argue with made-up stories
• Respond to the person's feelings, not their words
• Use distractions
• Do not try to reason with the person
• Give yourself permission to alter the truth for your loved one's sake
• Avoid asking questions that rely on memory
• Break down all tasks into simple steps
• Respond calmly to anger; don't contradict.
• Try to stay relaxed and SMILE.

For additional information or to request a copy of Compassionate Care and Communication: Best ways to interact with the person with dementia, contact the Alzheimer's Association Orange County Chapter at 800.272.3900. Alzheimer's Association Orange County Chapter, rev. 2012

To: Rhonda
From: Carolyn

This was in the book I found at the Library! So helpful to see this again. Can't believe I'm actually getting permission to lie to my mom and it has an official name. Therapeutically fibbing to my mother. You have no idea...

And so I regaled Fay with stories about the vacation she was on for the summer and how much fun we were going to have, and that she could go home whenever she decided. And I looked her in the eyes the entire time with a straight face, forcing myself to take steady breaths.

Our first evening in Mom's new house felt absurdly uncomfortable, and the air crackled with wire tight tension. Neither Roxanne nor I knew the right thing to say if Mom asked us any details about her trip there or the reason all her things were in this new house. We had little practiced scripts in our heads for some possible scenarios, but our mother had a way of shooting zingers we couldn't dodge. Each time she brought up her house in Georgia (and sometimes she flashed all the way back to New York), Roxanne's eyes would dart over to me and one of us would commence with our script.

Light conversation quickly turned into quicksand, and since neither of us knew when we might step into it, we stopped talking altogether. We made a light dinner from the groceries I'd brought over earlier and ate in silence. The only sound in the kitchen after dinner was the clinking of dishes as I washed and Roxanne dried. We hung back while our mother looked around the house a little more before I hinted it was time for me to go to my own home and get some sleep.

Mom surprised me by following me to her bedroom and allowing me to take a nightgown out of her dresser for her. She was clearly exhausted from traveling and the introduction to her new home. I tucked her into bed and went out to the living room to find my sister sitting on the edge of the couch waiting for me. She looked terrified. She asked me not to leave her in the house alone with Mom, which sent shivers through me as I realized we were both petrified of her.

I could've stayed. Shared the bed with her. Instead I reassured her that Mom was dead tired and already asleep in her room, gave her a quick hug, and slinked out the front door. I couldn't drive away fast enough.

I returned the next morning with breakfast burritos and

orange juice to find Fay in the kitchen, every cabinet door open as she busily rummaged through them. She didn't look up or acknowledge me when I called out, just continued removing pots and pans and setting them on the countertops and floor.

"Look at this! They have all my things!"

Roxanne pulled me into the bathroom to tell me that she was awakened sometime in the night by a noise in her room. When she turned on the light, she caught Mom right as she was getting ready to pee in her closet.

I know I mentioned that my sister and I weren't really close but having her there with me those two days was like having a security blanket I never wanted to put down. She was the buffer between my mom and me. I didn't want to be left alone with my own mother – what did that say about me? I felt like a monster inside, hiding this secret I didn't say out loud. But the fact that I couldn't predict her next move left me constantly on edge and off balance. By now I'd seen enough to know that whatever she delivered, it was going to be full of accusations that would make navigation tricky; and she was surely going to trip me up in a lie.

My sister was already due back at work, and knowing she was about to leave me unleashed a fresh wave of dread through my body. I knew she had no choice, but I felt like she was abandoning me, and I resented her for having such an iron clad excuse to leave. Now I was going to have to manage my mother *without* any backup.

You would think that our mother would be upset with Roxanne's impending departure – some emotional outburst that one of her daughters was leaving her in this strange place. But even as my sister popped her last things into her suitcase while we sat on the bed watching, Mom's only focus was squeezing one of Grandma's quilts in there as a gift. She told us how her mother had sewn one for her each time they brought one of us home from the adoption agency. I'd never heard that story, but she sounded earnest, and who knew?

So with a bulging suitcase and two sweatshirts tied around her waist, my sister hugged our necks and was out the door. I imagined she must have felt like she'd been sprung from jail and couldn't wait to get back home. And just like that, Fay and I had been deserted, left together in her new little house, both feeling a little uneasy and very awkward.

Robert offered to drive my sister to the airport while I stayed with Mom, since there was no way I was putting her back in that car with us for another miserable five hour round trip. I certainly couldn't leave Robert alone with her (he was just as unnerved by the idea as I was). She'd been particularly short with him for some reason, and the sweeter he was to her, the nastier she got. He could be hovering near the kitchen table and offer, *"Fay, can I get you another cup of coffee?"* and she'd clip, *"You know I don't drink coffee,"* empty coffee cup in front of her. So it was decided that I'd stay behind.

We spent the day browsing through her new yard and discovering all the plants and early spring flowers just beginning to sprout. We managed two walks around the neighborhood to kill some more time, me pointing at pretty houses and her commenting on newly budding trees. The unseasonably warm day had coaxed everyone out into their yards as Idaho springs do, and she met quite a few of her curious new neighbors (folks she would continue to "meet" repeatedly over the next several months). She didn't like that they welcomed her to the neighborhood. And she particularly didn't like when they told her they'd been expecting her. Who were these sneaky people, and why were they all watching her? Still, she smiled politely and shook many hands as I introduced her to friends and acquaintances, many of whom would come to play key roles in keeping my mother safe.

We returned to the house after each outing, stepped through the front door, and the entire scene unfolded exactly as it had our first night. *"These look like my things! How did they get them here?!"* (I suppose she believed she was standing in *"their"* house and *"they"* had conspired against her to put them there.)

I didn't hesitate as I launched into my well-rehearsed script, reminding her she was visiting me for the summer and could go home any time she liked. Dale would put in for his vacation time at work and drive out to get her, just say the word. I learned quickly that the more details I gave, the more questions she fired back.

"What will happen to my garden?"

- Your neighbor is watering it.

"Who'll watch my house?"

- Dale is watching it.

"Who'll pay my bills?"

- (as if...) I've handled all your bills.

"Where's my car?"

(That one was a little trickier, since she wasn't getting it back, and I hadn't quite gotten the hang of fabricating stories on the fly.)

- It's in the shop. You hit something, and it needs to be repaired. (Don't blink, remain calm.)

Just when I thought I was getting rather good at it, she got me.

"Where's my green canister vacuum?" (You mean the one I threw into the 2nd roll-off dumpster?)

- It must be around here somewhere. We'll keep an eye out for it.

"No, I've looked everywhere. It's not here!"

- We'll keep looking. (Shhhhh... brain... hold steady... don't look away.)

That vacuum cleaner had been with me throughout my childhood. I'd killed countless butterflies in it, dropping them into the latch lid canister and letting them flutter around inside, hoping to re-dust their wings after I'd carried them around in my sweaty cupped hands for an afternoon. It had also quit working sometime later during my teenage years.

By late afternoon she'd forgotten about the green vacuum cleaner and had moved on to more dangerous territory. Where was Grandma's prized pinwheel quilt? *(You mean the one you crammed into Roxanne's suitcase this morning?)* The way she could remember the intricate history of a quilt but forget that she'd just stuffed it into her daughter's bag upset me more than it befuddled me. My logical mind screamed that she was trying to trick me. She was only pretending to be off balance! But I could tell from her confused expression that she wasn't fooling around. It would've broken my heart if I hadn't been so busy batting back the fire balls she hurled at me, still not fully believing she could've already forgotten what she did with that quilt.

Her pitch rose as she insisted someone had been in the house while we were out walking and stolen Grandma's quilt. She became more agitated as she countered each one of my recollections of the morning's quilt-cramming with, *"Why would I ever do that?!"* She simply refused to believe she put any quilt into Roxanne's suitcase, and I was utterly, emotionally spent. Every inch of me screamed to get out of that house.

Completely out of ideas about a different way to handle the mystery of the missing quilt, I scrambled for a believable story about why I needed to leave instead. I hoped my practical mother would fall for the distraction readily and without protest. Something work-related like laundry or going to the grocery store. I was so nervous that I could feel sweat trickling from my armpits down my sides. I took a deep breath and blurted, *"Well Mom, I'm going to go home now and do some chores. I'll see you in the morning."*

I'd bought her this nifty telephone with large number

pads. Each pad had a slot where you could insert a photo. Once programmed, all you needed to do was press the photo of the person you wanted to call, and it dialed their complete phone number.

"Here's the phone, Mom, and remember, all you have to do is push the button with my photo to call me."

She turned to me, startled, *"You don't live here, too?"*

Another tennis ball came whizzing past my head. *"I live right down the street in my own house,"* I said. *"Well, you can spend the night here with me."* Whoosh. Right by me again. *"I've got to do some work at my place tonight,"* I chirped. *"I'll see you first thing in the morning, and we'll have breakfast together. Give me a hug goodbye."* And off I sailed through the front door and straight out to my truck. Door closed, motor running, I glanced at the front picture window and there she stood, limp arms at her side like a deflated little bird. *I was two people in that moment. One who wanted to run back inside and sit with her all night, talking and drinking tea, and one who didn't even want to come back in the morning.*

She didn't come to the door when I knocked the next day, so I let myself in. I surveyed the room, and my first thought was that she'd been burglarized. Then I noticed that everything was still there – it had just multiplied by three and was scattered everywhere. Boxes, packing paper, bubble wrap, and every single item that hadn't gotten unpacked but HAD made it into her basement, was now UP from the basement and occupying the living room.

"Mom?" I called out, as I walked toward the formerly latch-locked door that was supposed to hide the basement stairs from her. *"Down here!"* she singsonged. I could feel my throat tighten. Rhonda was right – it was just a matter of time before she'd found that latch lock and finagled it open. We were so sure she'd never notice it at the very top of the door, and she certainly wouldn't be able to reach it. Wrong and

wrong. She'd just opened a gateway down treacherous stairs into a forbidden part of the house that was too late to take back now.

And these weren't your average stairs. They were twice as steep with treads half as deep. Even the most able-bodied user risked tumbling down them with one unfortunate foot misplacement. Add to that the regrettably placed electric panel box midway down the stairs that required you to bend forward and duck your head to half your height in order to avoid getting a good whap, and you've got yourself a potential disaster. My day had barely begun, and I was already in what was to become a routine state of dread by the time I reached the bottom step.

More boxes and paper littered the floor. I followed the chaos to the far room where everything had originally been stacked and there she was, grinning like a cartoon cat with a giant enamel canning pot in her arms, humming some non-tune.

"Look what I found!" she sang.

"I see that. Why don't we keep it down here until we have some canning to do?"

She nodded her head yes, eyes wide open and glassy, but she didn't release her grip on the pot as I led her toward the staircase. When I offered to hold it so she could go ahead of me, she snatched it away from my out-stretched arms and scooted up the flight of stairs, hunkered over her prize and humming.

I still remember my overwhelming sense of hopelessness as I followed her up. I was completely lost over what to do next or how to fix it so this wouldn't happen again. The basement was off limits, and I would've cried to anyone, defeated by the utter failure of this carefully thought-out plan, had I a sympathetic ear right then. But I didn't have one, like I often didn't when I was left alone with my mother.

Upstairs was a disaster. My poor, poor new-and-improved-mini-Fay house. In just a few days it had regressed to the mess we found in Georgia, minus the fruit flies and ants. I looked around and collapsed down onto the floor – the couch was piled high with boxes, cookie jars, and crockpots. Every cabinet door in the kitchen hung wide open again with pots, pans, and dry goods scattered across the floor.

"Mom, there's just no room for all this stuff upstairs. Didn't the house look so much nicer with less junk in it?"

Maybe I shouldn't have said junk. Or maybe she was tired of being told *"No."* But my mother's face twisted in way I've never seen as she worked herself into a rage just then. *"No. No. No! No! No!!"* over and over, faster and shriller. *"I know what you're trying to do! You're trying to steal all my things! But they're MINE. Not yours! What has happened to you? You're not the girl I raised! I want to call Dale – I want him to come get me NOW."*

It was unnerving to hear and even scarier to see, her face contorted into someone I didn't recognize. Like we were both actors rehearsing some movie scene and the director told her, *"Think of the worst thing EVER and show me how totally distraught you can make yourself over it."* I didn't know what to do or how to respond, so I just sat there, glued to the floor. I gathered a handful of crumpled packing paper and began smoothing it across my lap, staying focused on the paper. I didn't make eye contact with her as she huffed around the room, touching her things and shifting them around. She drifted into the kitchen, and I could hear her clinking coffee cups. I could've laughed when she exited with two cups of coffee and offered me one, but I was still reeling from her tongue lashing.

I accepted the coffee and searched her face, but there was no trace of the monster I'd just seen five minutes earlier. We both sipped our coffee – her humming a nonsense tune on a bare corner of the couch, and me silent on the floor. She wouldn't let me move anything or return them to their boxes, but she *WOULD* eventually let me stuff the packing paper back inside and carry them, empty, to the basement.

Ten minutes after the last box was returned downstairs, we were sharing grilled cheese sandwiches for lunch as if none of that madness had just happened. She kept exclaiming, *"These are so good! I've never had these before. What are they called again?"* These were the times I would swear she was pulling my leg. But that's not how it was with Fay; never any leg pulling. So another tennis ball came zinging toward my head as I tried to channel some of the advice from one of my books. I chose the sincere route and just repeated my answer as often as she asked, *"These are my special grilled cheese sandwiches. I'm kind of full, would you like the other half of mine?"*

I came back for dinner that evening and brought hamburgers and fries from Zip's Burgers, another treat for my mom and something I certainly was never raised with. When she met me at the door, she had the same look on her face as when I'd found her that morning in the basement. Kind of manic, with glassier eyes than a person should have, and a beyond normal smile plastered across her face. My stomach fell.

Every single emptied box I'd just hauled down to the basement that morning was back upstairs, scattered across the living room and dining room, packing paper everywhere.

"What happened, Mom? Why did you bring all the empty boxes back up and reopen them?"

Her answer: *"I wanted to make sure there was nothing inside."*

That's how it went, three meals a day with Fay while trying to pack as much into my personal life as I could between trips to her house. Most mornings I woke up with a pit in my stomach that I tried to talk myself past. I'd drink my coffee but hold off on breakfast until I got to Mom's. I could count five deep breaths as I made my way between my truck and her front door, forcing a sense of calm as I reached the front stoop. I'd never felt more alone, dreading what was in store for me inside.

She typically met me at the door before I even knocked. But on the mornings when she didn't answer and I had to look for her, I knew to begin in the basement. There she'd be, humming that same eerie tune, reopening boxes and arranging them on the floor, while another forgotten pot of beans scorched on the stove upstairs. Different from yesterday's scorched pot of beans sitting on the counter, and the scorched pot before that.

I was exhausted. It was Groundhog Day at Fay's house, and no amount of reasoning could keep her out of the basement, and her supply of dried beans was endless. I'd stopped lifting the lids to see what level of spoiled each pot was. I'd also started leaving the cabinet doors alone after several days of closing them. The kitchen looked like a scene from the movie *Sixth Sense*, where every single cabinet door was hanging open after the poltergeist had come through. I could only guess that she couldn't remember what was behind them, so this was her way of seeing what was there.

Same story with the refrigerator. There was a fresh gallon of milk on the counter, sweating next to a bloated gallon from the day before, and a near-bursting gallon from the day before that. How many times did I confront her about the milk? How many times did I return the newest gallon to the refrigerator? And how many times did she spray sour milk all over herself when she unscrewed the cap from the bloated container on the counter? This wasn't a onetime occurrence. This happened every day. And after she finished wiping up the milk, did she think to open the refrigerator and retrieve the fresh gallon? No, she tied up her laces and raced down the hill to the grocery store for another and the whole scene would begin again.

Every day at lunchtime I'd ask Mom what she'd like, anticipating her standard retort that there was no food in the house because I'd left her there without any. Not missing a beat, I'd open the fridge, begin pulling out food, and ask if she'd like a chicken sandwich, grilled cheese, soup... Her reaction was always the same, *"Oh! I didn't know that was in there!"*

I wish I could say my responses to my mother were as full of humor then as I write them down now. They weren't, though, and I regret this the most of all my sins. It was "the early days," when she was more lucid than she was not, and I was completely ill-prepared for times when she became lost. She was with it just enough to carry on believable conversations with only a smattering of strange. So when the strange came, it was incredibly unnerving, unpredictable, and unbelievably frustrating.

I couldn't seem to grasp the reality that she had a legitimate disease affecting her thoughts and actions beyond her control, like she had a Gremlin rambling around in her brain. I just wanted her to stop it. I wanted her to quit asking me the same question seven times in ten minutes. I wanted her to stop swearing that every new person she met had evil intentions toward her. And I especially wanted her to see that I wasn't the colossal disappointment she was convinced I was. She was impossibly difficult to love during those early days, and I gave in to that mindset more than I overcame it.

I remember thinking how impossible it would've been for my father to understand what was happening to my mother, and how relieved I was that he'd died before her symptoms presented themselves. There was no way, ever, he would have been able to cope with what was happening to her, and equally no way he would have been able to forgive the behaviors she couldn't now control. It made me sad to admit that I recognized the depth of understanding that was missing in their relationship, and I wondered how many other couples suffered the same way.

At some point during those days, she started feeling less like my mother and instead more like my responsibility, if that makes sense. Every day I would walk through her front door, soaked with anxiety and unprepared for what she had in store for me, but my profound need to keep her safe ensured my steady trips back to her house. It began to dawn on me that I'd singlehandedly built myself a prison. How naïve I had been, thinking that plucking my mother up and out of her environment and moving her closer to me would end her bizarre behavior. Instead, it simply guaranteed my title as both inmate and watchful guard in charge of preventing my own escape. I can honestly say that I've never felt more trapped and despondent than I did in those early days.

How many times did I cringe when a friend or simple acquaintance commented on my level of devotion to my mother? This, followed by what a loving daughter I must be. I felt like a monumental fraud, sure that my forced smile would betray me in my reaction to their compliment. I was a lot of things then – steadfast, thorough, dedicated – but loving daughter wasn't one of them. I felt truly little love then.

I remember taking my mother to my bank one day to open her own checking account. We stopped first at the sheriff's office to acquire a state ID for her since we never did find her driver's license, and I'd learned that by obtaining a state ID she could open her own account. Now she'd see proof of her $77 pension check deposits on her monthly statements and stop accusing me of robbing her of them. At least that was my hope.

The process was short, and within minutes she was being handed her very own checkbook. As we stood to leave our banker's desk, my arm tucked into hers to help her up, he reached over to shake her hand, saying, *"You're lucky to have such a loving daughter who wants to see that you're taken care of in your new home."*

She smiled her reply, *"Yes, and now I'll be able to catch her stealing from me red-handed."*

Still, there were days when her memory was clear, and her disposition was sweet. It was my mother! I saw her with my own eyes! I couldn't predict when I'd get a glimpse of her, or how long she would stay, but I found myself searching for her every time I came through the front door. It was as if Mother Nature had devised a way to protect my mother by encouraging my repeat visits with small and randomly placed rewards, just enough to keep me hopeful and returning – even after the most savage visits.

On a good day, she would beam as she recalled stories about our family and my childhood as if she hadn't just torn me to shreds with a biting snipe about my plan to bankrupt her and abandon her in an institution. A loving recollection would pop into her brain out of nowhere, and she'd tell me a story about how she met my father, or the time I carried a fish on the end of my pole all day and wouldn't let anyone touch it because it was my first.

And then minutes later, she was rifling through her desk because someone had clearly stolen all her pens. My mother was gone again, and this foreign version was seated in front of me, declaring I'd given away her favorite shoes.

If I had known how soon I was about to lose the stories, I swear I would've taken much greater care in retrieving as many as I could from her and savoring what was left. I swear.

I'll tell anyone now to take that drive down memory lane with your loved one as often as you can. Let them repeat their stories over and over. There might be a new tidbit in there you hadn't heard yet. Write it down. Ask for details. Because believe me, you'll have no idea when their last story is about to be told and no others will be following. You can't get them back, and the enormity of that is impossible to understand until it happens to you.

My "AA" Meetings.

I made so many mistakes over the next few months, but I read the books and continued to practice diversionary tactics with a quiet voice wherever I could. In between my numerous blunders with unfortunate outcomes, I witnessed the positive, promised results, and I began to settle myself into this new life with my confused, confrontational, and often pretty nasty mother.

Sometime that summer I spotted an Alzheimer's Association Meeting notice posted on the community board at the library. They were held at noon every first and third Thursday at the Panhandle Health building and co-hosted by two lovely women named Jolle and Carol. I walked into my first meeting, and I think I was crying within ten minutes. There may have been five of us, and they had just started sharing around the table when I sat down. I realized immediately that I was listening to stories just like mine. I mean, some of the exact same stories! For what felt like the first time since I moved Mom here, I was surrounded by people going through the same thing I was. I wasn't imagining things, I wasn't irrational (at least not entirely), and I certainly wasn't alone. It did take several rounds of hearing, *"You're not a terrible daughter; you're doing everything you can for her,"* to sink in.

I remember leaving that first meeting feeling wrung out and spent. I wasn't sure whether they'd be able to help me with the mechanics of "fixing Mom," but I knew I'd found a group of people to share my horrors with who knew exactly what I was experiencing, and who didn't try to give me advice clearly unsuited for my situation.

I dubbed them my "AA Meetings" and I made it to nearly every one that summer.

To: Carolyn
From: Jolle

It was so nice to meet you! Thank you for sending the link to the article in the Alzheimer's newsletter. It looks interesting and helpful. How is your mom handling the move these days? If you have time, I'd like to hear from you. Take good care of yourself.

To: Jolle
From: Carolyn

Thanks so much, Jolle, I really appreciate your email! Things are okay. Right now she's busy removing everything from each drawer and putting it somewhere else in the house. I don't know what that is or how to handle it. Today she told me, "My own daughter chooses to live in her own place when she could be living with her mother – just like a stranger." (This, after her insistence to live in her own house or she wouldn't come). That one led to a blow-up but thankfully it was over in five minutes and we made chili together. :-) Can't wait for the next meeting!

To: Carolyn
From: Jolle

I hope your mom is settling in okay. My mom moved everything from drawers too. Do you think it's because they want to be "busy" and that's all they can think to do? It sure makes it hard to do anything in the kitchen when you never know where anything will be! Is she content living alone? At some point it becomes dangerous for them. I know this isn't easy for you. Too bad your sister couldn't have stayed longer. Let me know how **you** are coping. I like hearing from you. Concerned.

To: Jolle
From: Carolyn

She likes to surround herself with her things, I do know that. It's like she's "safe keeping" by moving things, but then she can't remember where she put them. I wish I knew. I've noticed she can't "see" what she has unless it's out in plain view. She doesn't know she has crackers if they're in the pantry unless I take them out. Same with the refrigerator. Anything that gets put in there doesn't get eaten because she doesn't think to open the door. It's always, "Oh! I didn't know that was in there."

You know the story about Sondra tormenting her in Georgia by coming into her home at night and moving things around? That's come to an abrupt end. Incredible. How did Sondra disappear so suddenly? So far, no one's getting blamed when things have been "moved around." But I think my turn is next.

I just found out about the Senior Companion Program! Signing her up tomorrow. Penny from our Health Department is helping me sign her up for new supplemental Medicare insurance (her old supplement isn't serviced in this county). I never did find her Medicare card, but Penny thinks she can help me get a replacement and avoid driving to the office in Coeur d'Alene. I tried to do it myself by pretending to be Fay on the phone, but some of the information I entered didn't match what they had. Penny still thinks she can get me through to a person. She's incredible!

I'm already worried about leaving her alone and she's only been here a few months. I've found her stove burners on twice now. Someone suggested I disconnect the oven. She'd be furious! Trying to lay low and not interfere too much. She's super sensitive when I do anything. She's been calmer these past two days. "Where's my this?" and "Where's my that?" has slowed down a lot.

I enjoy hearing from you, too.

Over the course of several meetings, I found help with my mother's lost Medicare card through a patient advocate at the hospital. I was encouraged to seek Power of Attorney sooner than later, since I'd begun paying my mother's bills and no one would speak with me about any of her accounts without one. I learned how it works to sign up for assisted living if the need should arise, and I could see that the group was gently nudging me in that direction.

But most helpful of all (and I wish this were required continuing education for all caregivers), was the Alzheimer's Association DVD we watched of Teepa Snow's "Positive Approach to Care, Teaching Caregiving Techniques to Successfully Navigate Through Dementia-Driven Situations." Mother, husband, sister, grandparent – everyone could learn something from watching this.

> **To:** Carolyn
> **From:** Jolle
>
> How are you doing? Did you ever find the bananas? So many incidents since then you've probably forgotten the lost bananas. Let me know how you're managing. I hope your mom is happy in her new home and not making it too difficult for you. It's a hard time for you, I know.

> **To:** Jolle
> **From:** Carolyn
>
> Thank you so much for checking in! Every day is definitely different. She's teaching me so much and doesn't even realize it. Empathy instead of mean retorts. Her forgetfulness is eye-opening and humbling. One thing you said in the last meeting has stayed with me...*"You're never in front of this. You're always behind it trying to pick up the pieces."* Do you remember saying that? I'll bring some stories to the next meeting, but I'll bet you've already experienced each one.

That same summer I signed up for a "Living with Stress" seminar at our local health clinic. Just $89 and six weeks of my Monday, Wednesday, and Friday afternoons and I'd be better able to manage the stresses in my life. My willingness to sacrifice three treasured afternoons a week for six full weeks should speak volumes about my level of desperation. I'm sure the program was a huge help to many, but I knew almost immediately that I needed faster, more noticeable results than this class was going to give. I was drowning.

Classes began on Monday and opened with a mindfulness exercise involving eating a raisin. But we didn't eat the raisin. We looked at it. We smelled it. We squished it in our fingers. Then we were told to finally place it carefully on our tongues and keep it there while noticing its texture and sweetness and gentle plumping. The entire time I was supposed to be cultivating my mindfulness skills, I was instead thinking, *"When are we going to eat this freaking raisin!?"* That first exercise riled my frayed nerves as much as my mother could any day, and I was already doubting my decision to spend almost a hundred bucks on this class instead of a cool pair of shoes.

On Wednesday we formed a group circle and were asked to "share something positive to balance something negative" about our day. When it was my turn, I asked if I could pass. I wanted to be a team player and participate as guided, but my mom and I had already had a terrible morning, and I couldn't draw a single positive thing from the remainder of my day to balance that. I looked around our circle as my tears burbled near the surface, watching awkward glances flit between the people in the group and over to our leader. The thought of getting emotional in front of everyone paralyzed me as I held my breath, willing her to say, *"Okay, pass."*

Instead, she pressed me to share anyway, and "work through it with no judgment." I sat there, frozen. I took a deep breath and as I opened my mouth to speak, some animal sound eeped out instead. *I choked back a sob as my throat clenched so tightly that the sour taste of vomit filled the back of my mouth. Grabbing up my shoes at the door and hurrying toward the exit, I kept my eyes focused on the floor to avoid the stares of disbelief I knew I'd see if I looked up.* I could hear our leader's muffled voice in the background saying something about the importance of staying in class and being surrounded by our loving, supportive group as I heaved open the door and pitched through it to the reception area. My truck was parked right outside the classroom windows, and I could see everyone hovering nervously on the other side, peering through them as I backed out and drove away. It was our second day of class, and I never went back.

I'd been living for weeks like I'd been dumped into some cesspool and was trying hard not to swallow the sludge as I gulped for air. I was nearly at rock bottom, if that's a place you can recognize once you get there. I dreaded my morning alarm clock because it signaled a new day that began with a trip to my mother's. My world had shrunk to within a tiny radius around Fay's house.

I'd even stopped driving to our neighboring town where the nearest Home Depot and Starbucks were because I was afraid the seventy-mile round trip would be too far for me to hurry back when the next panic call came. My outings were reduced to grocery shopping and the post office, and even those were littered with dangerous emotional land mines. Someone would invariably stop me to ask about my mother, I'd try for some simple, upbeat response, and somehow end up in a very public crying jag.

But the universe really does work in mysterious ways, and slowly little glimpses of relief began to show themselves, reassuring me that I was surrounded by help, guidance, and love. Two steps forward and all that, but things were quietly beginning to fall into place and problems started working themselves out. Right around the time of my stress management class meltdown, I received my annual pap smear reminder. I hadn't thought about it since last year (probably the reason they make your next annual appointment for you before you leave). Maybe it was good that I'd quit my "Living with Stress" seminar – at least I didn't have to miss their next class for my GYN appointment and get all stressed out about it.

My patient workup that day was uneventful. I was weighed – down 10 lbs. from last year, Yay! – blood pressure taken – *"Hmm... it's higher than normal, did you run here?"* And the usual questions – *"No, no real changes in my life since last year. No complaints. No unusual circumstances that might be of concern,"* as I sat there shivering in my paper gown. My doctor came in and shook my hand, then looked over the nurse's notes. *"You've lost some weight since last year and your blood pressure is higher than customary; is anything going on in your life that may be contributing to these changes?"*

I swear to God, I opened my mouth to say that I didn't think so when I took a shuddering breath and heaved out an explosive sob. This wasn't the crying-with-tears kind of sobbing, but more like the snot-shooting-out-my-nose-and-choking-on-my-own-spit-as-I'm-trying-to-catch-my-breath kind of sobbing. It took several minutes to slow myself down while she instructed me through some steady breathing exercises. *"Wow, I didn't see that coming,"* I croaked, and we both laughed, which helped me release a little more. When I was able to form complete sentences, I told her everything, from the sheriff's phone call all the way to whatever frightening thing my mother had done that morning.

And *that* was the day I learned about Caregiver's Stress Syndrome and situational Prozac. It was also the day I decided that situational Prozac might be for me, which is saying a lot for a girl who balks at taking an ibuprofen. I walked out of my annual GYN appointment without a breast exam, pap smear, or even pelvic exam, but I *DID* have one small square of paper in my hand that filled me with hope, "Fluoxetine 20 mg – take one every morning for six months, 0 refills." I beelined to the pharmacy. I did not pass GO, and I did not collect 200 dollars.

I signed where instructed, paid my $10 co-pay, and swallowed TWO pills in the parking lot with the cold stale coffee in my console.

To: Rhonda
From: Carolyn

Guess who's got a prescription for Prozac??? I don't even know what to do with myself! Am I going to get better now or am I some weakling who just can't handle it? My doctor wrote the script this morning and I've already taken two. There's a website called caregiver.com and if you type in "caregiver's stress syndrome" in the search bar, you can read all about me.

GIVE ME BACK MY MOTHER!

There are other stories I should tell, like the day Robert and I were driving to Sandpoint and he pointed at a lady speed-walking along the highway, hat pulled down tight on her head and bent over the weight of her grocery bag, and laughed, *"That looks just like Fay."* And of course, it was.

He swung the truck off the highway and stopped it just beyond her line of sight so she wouldn't see us as we inched forward to keep up with her as she scooted along. We were both shocked that she'd made it this far from home – at least a mile! Neither of us could've predicted that this would be something we'd have to consider – Fay on the highway – AND she'd crossed over to the other side somewhere along her route.

We debated whether we should let her make it home on her own or stop the madness and pick her up now. He with, *"Let's get her before she steps in front of a car,"* and me with, *"But what will I say when she starts screaming at me?"*

I wasn't feeling ready for the new round of tennis balls I knew she'd serve up: *"Why are you following me?"* *"Take me home! (to Georgia, maybe New York)"* *"Where do I live again?"* and I was still a newbie with dementia-dealing, so every fresh, scary question sent me into a tailspin.

While we sat there considering what to do, a car pulled up alongside her, its window rolled down, and just like that Mom popped into the back seat as they eased into traffic. It happened exactly that fast, and all we could do was stare. We tried to follow closely behind so we could flash our lights and

91

signal them to pull over, but we'd become separated by several cars. I began to panic, which didn't help us with our couple's calm decision-making skills practicing. My phone rang just then with a number I didn't recognize, and I did my best not to sound hysterical as I answered to the people who had my mother. A very timid man hesitatingly introduced himself, explained that he and his wife were traveling north to Canada from Boise, and launched into a slow, detailed story about how they had just picked up this elderly lady on the highway and were wondering if...

How do you stay composed during a time like this? I'd just suffered five mini heart attacks after catching my mother walking on this new stretch of highway, on the wrong side no less. And while fighting with Robert over whether to snatch her up or leave her be, she climbs into a stranger's car. Now add the fact that we couldn't catch up with the car that in my mind was taking her off to her most certain and tortured death. *"Of course I know who this is and the story you're stammering to get out! Now please pull over and give me back my mother!"* Of course I didn't say any of this, realizing the need to sound normal and appreciative – which I was, appreciative. Probably not so normal.

Luckily, I had written my name and number on my mother's house keys, recommended to me by my new friends at my Alzheimer's meetings, and that's how this nice couple found me. That bit of advice had proved to be invaluable more than once. Fay would be out scouting and regularly become lost. She could never recount for anyone where exactly she lived, but somehow she always knew to take out her key ring to show them she did indeed live somewhere, and there they'd see my name and number in neon.

Mom's "highway travel" was particularly disconcerting because we had taken great pains to show her the route DOWN the hill into town, all left turns and no highway crossings, to the LITTLE grocery store where I'd already introduced her to the staff and opened a "Fay Account" so she would never be turned away without her groceries if she were short of cash. We weren't prepared for her to turn RIGHT.

> **To:** Ginny
> **From:** Carolyn
>
> Mom got into a FREAKING CAR today! And she was on the highway! Don't ask me why she decided to turn right this time, but we spotted her all the way down by the car wash on the south end of town on our way to Home Depot just as someone was pulling over to pick her up. She just jumped in! They called me within minutes. A nice couple who had her in their back seat – they thought she looked out of place on the highway with a grocery bag so they stopped. Lucky!

> **To:** Carolyn
> **From:** Ginny
>
> OMG! She's never turned right before, has she? Isn't this like the third time someone's called you from her keychain? What are you going to do now?

> **To:** Ginny
> **From:** Carolyn
>
> I don't know. How do I stop her now that she's discovered a whole new world to the right?

Neither of us knew how, but this was a problem we needed to solve immediately, because now that she'd discovered this whole new world, she was going to want to see more of it. But right now, I was simply happy to have her out of that car and safely in her home. Just like that grease fire, I stamped it out and hoped it would be the last.

Up or down the hill, Fay was going to walk. There was no way I could stop her from shooting out her door at any time of the day. It became a regular occurrence to see her heading to or from downtown, followed by a call or two from some well-intentioned person letting me know Fay was "out for her walk."

I had to make peace quickly with the fact that she could and would walk as far as her legs would carry her. I couldn't lock her in her house, and I couldn't be with her every minute of the day. In fact, she developed a routine of waiting until I was *just* pulling out of her driveway – I would watch for her in my rearview mirror – and out she would spring from the front door, screwing her hat down onto her head and darting toward the hill. I could only imagine her feeling of liberation for having pulled one over on me by escaping the lockdown I had surely imposed on her.

Sometimes she'd do this after breakfast AND lunch. Those were the days I'd find TWO gallons of room temperature milk on the counter when I stopped by for dinner. Some days I'd get the call that "Fay was out walking," and I'd intercept her, asking if I could join her. She'd screw up her face and say, *"I'm walking to the store because you left me in the house without any food." "And what did you do with my car?" "I shouldn't have to walk in this heat!" "When can I go home?" "I want to call Dale."* I'd step in line with her and begin practicing my budding deflection skills.

Some days I'd do better than others and manage to change the subject, get her to tell me a story, and coax a smile out of her. Other days I'd quietly walk alongside her and count the minutes until we made it back to the house. And at some point on our walk we'd often run into someone I knew and I'd introduce them to my mother, who'd respond with, *"Yes, I'm her mother. She leaves me alone in the house with no food. AND she stole my car."*

FRIENDS, FAMILY, AND FACEBOOK –
BUT STILL IN OVER MY HEAD.

I think it was the Alzheimer's group who helped me see that with as much progress as I had made, and with as many resources as I had found, I was still in over my head. My crying outbursts had diminished, but my Fay stories grew.

Or maybe it was Robert who said it; poor thing, he was suffering as much as I was, only his was from *my* abuse – Fay fallout – while I remained in first position, getting it directly from the source. Sadly, almost everything he offered was received by me as a criticism. I felt like he thought I was doing everything wrong. Every solution he offered sounded to me too cold and unfeeling to deliver from a daughter to her mother. *"You should tell her she can't turn right onto the highway; she's going to get hit by a car." "You shouldn't give her any more cash so she can't buy anything from the store; she's wasting it anyway." "Tell her she can't go down into the basement anymore because she might fall down the stairs."*

If I had friends struggling to deal with a loved one's dementia, I'd suggest they over communicate with each other and start their sentences with something like, *"It must be so hard to make this decision for your mother/ father/ grandmother... but what if we tried (insert here) together and see how it goes?"* Nothing feels as disparaging as when your partner issues directives on how you should be doing something that is clearly different from what you are currently doing. When your nerves are already frayed and all you hear is criticism about your management style toward your loved one, who clearly isn't responding the way you've intended either, it leaves you doubting your own decision making, and open, loving communication flies right out the window.

Maybe it was the breath of clarity I'd begun to feel from the Prozac hidden deep in my drawer – the dirty shame I swallowed faithfully every morning as though it were keeping me alive. Or maybe it was every new incident that seemed to get a little worse each time. Wherever it came from, it was finally clear to me that I needed more help. That's when I truly turned to my family, friends, and social media.

From my family, help came from my sister, who sympathetically listened as I lined up my Fay stories like tin soldiers. She always answered her phone when I called, which I recognized was a special consideration, since her days were filled with speedy mail deliveries and constant public interaction.

I remember calling her one day, crouched on the far side of my truck in Mom's driveway so she couldn't see me from her window, unable to form words while choking back sobs. I'd had to step outside after Mom had finished telling me what a filthy liar I was (her words) for stealing her pension checks from her, and what a huge regret I was to her. Roxanne just waited on the other end of the line until I was quiet and told me how sorry she was that I was going through this alone. She *knew* our mother and was as incredulous as I was. She felt sorry *with* me, and that was exactly what I needed. She didn't tell me this disease was cruel and that it wasn't really our mother saying those things. Because it really *was* her saying those things, and she meant every word, disease or no.

I think I struggled most with the conflict that coursed through me like the very blood my heart pumped. Our mother raised us to *never* say an unkind word to anyone. (Imagine growing up with two other siblings in a household where any sort of verbal sparring was banned!) Now here she was, slashing me open with her words. I loved her! I revered her. I even believed her. And I hated her. What I'm trying to say is she taught me *all* the things. She taught me kindness and compassion through her actions. Everything I know about hard work and frugality I learned from her. And to this day, I whisper, *"Sorry Mom,"* when I use my finger to help the last bit of food from my plate onto my fork.

So here I was, left to sort out this contradiction that was my mother. She hated me. But she didn't hate me. I was keeping her safe. But she swore abuse. I was caring for her. But she felt abandoned.

My friend Ginny, having her own strong interest in dementia-related behavioral issues, had begun asking about Fay and checking in on me. She had a close friend whose mother was exhibiting signs of dementia and had begun enlisting her help with daytime companion services. Ginny's own mother was starting to alarm the family with some scary behaviors as well, so we fell into comparing stories and bouncing ideas off each other pretty naturally. I think it was Ginny who offered to stop in and see Fay from time to time, just another set of eyes on her.

I remember my mixture of relief and guilt as I reassured her that Mom was easy, even pleasant. That no, she shouldn't worry about Mom slipping away from her or refusing to be led back home. At this point, I think I would've said anything to secure her help, and I figured I'd just deal with it if Fay got ornery and caused any problems. One more visit here and there from Ginny would feel like a mini vacation for me and I wasn't going to risk losing it.

The reality was Ginny had already heard the stories through my tears and was rightfully apprehensive about her first few trips to Fay's. But Mom took to her immediately and really *was* pleasant and easy to be with. Ginny's visits turned into regular walks, since it was a perfect way to work in a little activity, keep her mind occupied, and it was Fay's absolute favorite thing to do. I received regular email updates from her that were both a comfort and a source of comedic relief for both of us, I think. Our friendship was a casual one that grew a little more multi-faceted from being "comrades in battle." Much later, *I began to recognize and appreciate the many glasses of lemonade that would eventually be poured for me from all the lemons I'd been handed,* Ginny's friendship being one of them.

To: Carolyn
From: Ginny

I dropped in on Fay this afternoon, and all went very well. She seemed to be in good spirits and was good company. She's a feisty thing, isn't she? :) After about 15 minutes of conversation with her on her couch, I headed off to finish my walk, and she came with me! We just went around her block, and she showed me some "landmarks" she knew along the way. She told me several times that today she tried to get a perm at the Beauty Salon but they were closed. Then she showed me her wad of money and asked if I thought it was enough. (It was quite a wad!!) Just wanted to give you a heads up because I think she'll try for that perm again tomorrow. All in all (apart from a story in which her neighbors in Georgia robbed her of all her Hummels) she was a pleasure. Was she really married 3 times?

To: Carolyn
From: Ginny

Spent 20 minutes walking the neighborhood with Fay this afternoon. In today's "heads up" category – Fay locked herself out this morning. Rather than call you (which I strongly suggested, but *after* the fact) she went to her neighbors' house(s?) and the woman who lives in the blue house behind her cherry tree apparently came to the rescue in more ways than one – she called a locksmith AND whipped out her checkbook to pay the $40 fee when Fay stated she didn't have that kind of money (she certainly DID have that kind of money in the wad she showed me the other day). "Well then you *do* have very nice neighbors, Fay," I said, referring to her comment that she had bad neighbors the other day: You probably already have back-up lock out plans in place, but it unfortunately doesn't mean she'll follow them. Sorry, I know this falls in the "this sucks" category, and I questioned even telling you. I think Fay is just very invested right now in her independence. I don't know the neighbors' name, or even how true this story is, for that matter...

To: Ginny
From: Carolyn

Geesh! I hate hearing this, but please always tell me everything. I'll have to go find her neighbor to thank/pay her. And no, I didn't have a back-up lock out plan, but I do now!

Had to call the Schwann's man today. Found another big box of ice cream bars in her freezer. Plus she says she's out of money again!! I gave her $40 two days ago. It was a different guy this time who didn't know about her diabetes. I told him I wouldn't interfere yet, since she really enjoys his stops. But I will if it gets out of hand. He's going to tell her he's out of ice cream next time. I also told him to keep it under $20. She still has the three mystery candy bars on the counter. I snagged an unopened bag of miniature chocolates when she wasn't looking. We weeded the front yard together and I made her a grilled cheese sandwich for lunch. I brought fruit and $40 more. She's going through it every few days.

My friends Kim and her mother Betty also became regular audience members to the "Fay Follies." They owned a little resale baby clothes boutique right up the street from my mom's house. I had no baby to buy for, but I found myself stopping in to say hello on a fairly regular basis, and we usually ended up on the subject of my mother. Theirs was the sympathetic ear I needed, and Betty could relate from her days as an in-home caregiver. Plus they had a candy machine that dispensed Mike and Ikes, and I had plenty of quarters.

Betty offered to drop in on Fay sporadically as well, since

their store was close by. I tried the same line of reassurances I'd used on Ginny with Betty, but she stopped me short with, *"Carolyn, believe me when I say I've seen it all. I can take care of myself – you don't have to worry about me."*

I can't recall exactly if it's true, but if you asked Kim, she'd probably confirm that I cried pretty much every time I stopped by their shop with some new story about a particularly tough time with Mom, some so terrible that even Kim would tear up. Now, with Betty's added help, I had a glimpse of a pinprick of light at the end of the tunnel. She was the perfect solution in my eyes – practical, closer to my mother's age, and she already had experience with home healthcare.

I'll never know how connections are formed between two people, and especially not where my mother is concerned. But within just a few visits from Betty, my mother stopped answering her door when she dropped by. Then one day she snapped at me, *"That white haired woman only comes by because she wants my house."* And just like that, my newly forming army was being single-handedly picked off by my little mother. Note to self: Warn any future angels to avoid complimenting Mom on her house or any of the things in it.

With my friends and family fully utilized, I turned to Facebook out of simple desperation. I posted a photo of me and my mother in front of her house and introduced Mom as the town's newest resident. I provided her mailing address and invited my Facebook friends to send her a "welcome to the neighborhood" card. A genius idea! My mother had become fixated on the mailman ever since she moved in. He was a constant source of anxiety for her, never leaving anything in her box and obviously in cahoots with me as I intercepted her mail in my scheme to drain her of all her money. She'd either be at her front window at 11am waiting for a glimpse of him or wandering around outside near the mailbox if the weather was decent. Then she would hit that poor man with the same line of questioning as she had from the day before.

"Where have you been?"

– Uh... delivering mail, I guess.

"I haven't seen you in days."

– I was here yesterday, I promise.

"Do you have anything for me?"

– Not today, I'm sorry.

"Are you sure?"

– Yes, ma'am.

"Maybe you should check your bag."

– I double checked; I don't have anything for you.

"Do you know my daughter, Carolyn?"

– No, ma'am.

"She steals from me and keeps me locked inside."

– (Raised eyebrows.)

Within a few days, my mother began receiving mail! It was heartwarming to see her surprised face when the mailman personally handed her the first few envelopes – even he was smiling. She received lovely cards and short notes that were sent from all over the United States welcoming her and congratulating her on her new house. People wrote about how much her daughter loved her and that they couldn't wait to meet her. I was touched by the generosity of my friends, some merely acquaintances from whom I'd accepted a random friend request at some point.

But Fay's disposition changed from startled happiness to suspicious anger within one day. I stopped by the morning after her first mail delivery to find her sitting on the couch with about four cards and their envelopes spread out over her lap.

"Who is this card from? And how did she get my address?"

– She's that nice lady up the street who talks to you about her flowers every morning, Mom.

"That woman doesn't care about me! She just wants to get in my house, and now she knows where I live! YOU did this, didn't you!?"

She was seething and I was reeling. None of this made sense to her, and it definitely wasn't welcomed. All these people were watching her, and it was my fault.

It wasn't until the next day when Mom didn't answer the door that I realized my good intentions had backfired beyond my imagination. I let myself in to find her hunkered over her favorite coffee table, fanning the flames on a small pile of mail – a black layer of smoke wafted around the living room, choking me as I ran over to snuff out the fire.

"Mom! Why did you have to burn these cards?!"

- Because, NOW they can't find me.

How does burning cards erase the sender's knowledge of where someone lives? How could she see these lovely cards and letters as threats to her security? And where the hell did she find matches??

My AA Group had gotten more vocal about my need to begin investigating alternative care for my mother, and the matches story was met with alarm and a greater sense of urgency. With Betty no longer dropping in and Ginny only there a couple of times a week, I was still making three visits every day unless Ginny's timing was during lunch and I caught a break. The relief I'd hoped for hadn't arrived, and my mother possessed a healthy imagination as to what kind of trouble she could get into and how often.

It was beyond my comprehension how I was ever going to convince her to move into an assisted living situation, and she certainly wasn't going to allow a private caregiver into her home. I felt blocked on all sides. There simply wasn't a ready answer, and my options seemed nonexistent.

You could say that I continued to kick that can down the road. I coped by continually minimizing each new calamity and reassuring myself with that it would be the last, or that at least I could handle the next one so much better from whatever lesson I'd just learned. I actually stopped contributing "Fay stories" to the group with a vague, *"No, nothing new this week to report,"* because I didn't want to be pushed any further.

But the Fay stories continued to roll in. And they escalated.

Her new backyard had an enormous cherry tree, and it was late June, almost cherry season. Every day presented the possibility of ripe fruit, and for Fay, that meant sampling as many green cherries as her body could handle, in case they had ripened from the day before. I couldn't reason with her to leave them alone until they were ready, so I decided to take my AA group's advice and worry less about it. She wasn't suffering from any stomach distress and the only person upset by it was me.

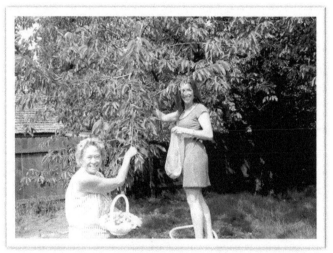

~ I probably planted the seed by using the step ladder ~

The latest book I was reading warned against trying to protect your loved one to the point of exhaustion (certainly mine) and let them find their own way. Since I seemed to be receiving the same advice from all directions, it made sense to take notice and maybe practice a little.

And then one day as if by miracle, the tree ripened, and we spent afternoons under it eating glorious fruit. With the lower branches emptied, though, my newest challenge began. I had to devise a way to keep that determined woman from standing on overturned buckets and chairs to get to the higher unpicked bounty. I'd managed so far by simply removing any buckets from the yard. The chairs in the house were too heavy for her to move without anyone to help her.

That next day I left her after we had lunch, but when I returned for dinner, she didn't answer the door. I let myself in and glanced around, calling her name. I moved toward the basement door and steeled myself for the mess I was about to discover, but it was silent down there, too. I peered out into the backyard from the kitchen window and saw nothing, so I decided to drive down the hill to look for her in the grocery store. I opened the door to my truck and reached for my seatbelt. That's when I heard the humming. I recognized the non-tune right away, and I knew it well enough by now to understand it meant trouble and tennis balls. I followed it into the backyard and spotted the Lazy-Boy recliner behind the cherry tree, but no Fay.

The humming resumed and I looked up. There she was, high in the tree. I mean, *"How the James Hill did she get that far up?"* kind of high. Getting her to lower herself down branch by branch was going to be perilous and slow going, which I was prepared for. I *wasn't* prepared for her to flat out refuse to come down. After a ridiculous amount of time spent trying to convince my glassy-eyed, humming mother to climb down with every logical reason I could conjure, I remembered an article I'd read about dealing with them on their new "level," and shouted up to her, four-year-old-style, *"Fine, you stay up there while I go inside and eat the fried chicken and mashed potatoes I brought you for dinner."* The chicken needed to be reheated by the time she was down, but she did come down.

$\mathcal{A}$NGELS ARE EVERYWHERE.

I believe in the notion that you don't really meet anyone by accident. People enter and exit our lives for very real reasons, and my friend Denise is all the proof I need. We met each other in morning step class at the gym. Our friendship began after many makeup-free hours spent sweating to thumping music and smart aleck comments about our butts. As new friends do, we began to share little things as we got to know each other. My little things happened to be centered around my mother, since she was occupying most of my thoughts those days. It must have touched something inside Denise, because when I told her one morning about Fay's latest escape down the highway, she offered to be her walking buddy without any hesitation or thought. She reasoned that she was an avid walker anyway and said it would be fun to stop by Fay's house and stroll around the block with her once or twice a week.

I'm telling you, *angels are everywhere, and I knew I'd just encountered one.* Once or twice a week turned into their "afternoon walks," and I suddenly found myself coordinating schedules between me, Ginny, and Denise. I finally felt like relief was in sight. I had my A-Team, I had Alzheimer's Association Meetings to attend, I had Robert, and even my ex-husband Sam – we were an awesome, if unlikely crew.

To: Carolyn
From: Denise

Today Fay and I talked, watched a little TV, watered her plants, and walked. Boy can she walk! I had to keep up!

Today the subjects were: her sister's untimely death in the middle of the night with telephone in hand, the same sister's stubborn husband who bought property on a mountain top and how he kept tripping on rocks, her neighbor stealing her garlic, Fay's former goat who was The Guest at a party, her fat Italian mother-in-law, and my poor decision not to have kids. She makes me laugh.

To: Denise
From: Carolyn

Such sad, confused thoughts. Aunt May was her twin. She died a few years ago from adult-onset diabetes – they were diagnosed the exact same month. But she didn't manage hers as strictly as Mom does. I know she misses her. We talked about you today and guess how old you are? 20 or 21. AND you have TWO KIDS. So there. No more poor decisions for you. That explains why Mom asked me in a very accusing way why I had asked her for Aunt May's address. I told her I never asked for it and she got really agitated, suspicious, and told me I was trying to trick her.

Now that visits were becoming much more regular, we agreed that everyone was going to get paid. This was much more than the generosity of friends, and I couldn't accept all their help without contributing in some way, and what better way than to pay them? They were Fay-sitters for Pete's sake! And I knew full well that they were going to earn it. I was amazed that I had to convince them to accept anything. They were each worth gold to me, which I didn't have, but we came up with agreeable terms, and the rest was history. Well, you know that thing about history.

I may have gotten an afternoon or morning break, but my mother's antics didn't lessen one bit, and so I was often called in to sweep up some mess she'd created when her behavior got a little too uncomfortable for Denise or Ginny. They'd either call or email me with "today's latest Fay-this or Fay-that." So the relief I had anticipated still hadn't come. If I got a glimpse of it for a day or two, I'd fool myself into believing things were calming down, sure again that she was going to be happy living in her cute little house nearby.

But two days was about the max before the proverbial "all Hell" broke loose, sending Ginny and Denise into a tailspin of uncertainty and me into the decision-maker role.

Still in recruitment mode, I turned to family for help once again, this time from my ex-husband Sam. We had moved to Idaho to retire from our real estate business and escape the home building craziness going on in Atlanta in 2006. Somehow we were lucky enough to make the move about five minutes before the bubble burst, but our ten-year marriage wasn't as lucky and dissolved barely six months later. My Atlanta girlfriends begged me to come home, unless, they said, I was bent on committing relationship suicide in my new town (population 2,500) and being single for the rest of my life.

But I stayed, met Robert, and found my way with Sam. We managed to become friends again and he stayed involved through the whole ordeal leading up to and including flying out to get my mother. I'd kept him in the loop, since he'd known her for over a decade, and was among the audience who heard my "hilarious Fay stories." He always stopped in on Mom whenever he came into town to get groceries, often bringing her something from his garden, and she loved that.

He regularly invited us out to his farm to pick raspberries or have lunch. Mom loved to feed his horses apples or throw scratch to his chickens. It was a nice diversion for her and something for us to do besides sit in her house. I remember one particularly lovely afternoon when we'd brought him a big container of white beans and sausage (from a fresh pot I'd supervised) and we made strawberry shortcake in his kitchen with the fresh berries from his garden. We sat on his porch afterward, watching a mama bird flit in and out of the bird house, tending to her new hatchlings.

That night my phone rang, and it was Sam. Before I could say hello, he said, *"You know you're not doing your mother any favors by keeping her in that house. You're basically the only one she sees, and three meals a day doesn't fill 24 hours. She's lonely and bored. No wonder she's getting into trouble and taking everything out on you."*

At a time when I was feeling uncertain about everything, he sounded so certain. All I could do was cry. (Gosh, I do cry!) Not over the fact that he'd easily made a clear assessment that I seemed incapable of making, but from relief that a solution was being presented that I hadn't been ready to consider until just that moment.

He made it seem so simple! Mom plainly needed to be in an assisted living situation where she would have more people to interact with and certainly more eyes on her. It was time to let go of everything I'd been trying to accomplish up until now.

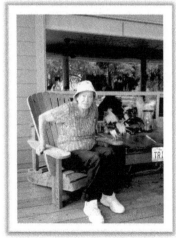

~ *Mom with Buddy,*
Sam's rooster ~

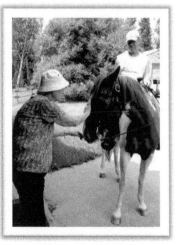

~ *She was so tentative,*
yet gentle! ~

But even as the light bulb went off, I knew I was going to need a whole lot more help with the execution. How on God's green earth was I going to manage this? She still had a healthy ability to say *"no,"* and used it often. She had two perfectly good legs to walk out any door she decided. And she could she cut me off at the knees with her flat-out refusal to do something, not to mention her anger over my suggestion in the first place.

I brought it up at my next AA meeting and was unanimously encouraged to proceed, no matter how difficult it was going to be. It finally felt like the right thing to do, and I was resolved to begin planning this next move. And I was terrified.

To: Carolyn
From: Denise

Dropped in on Fay today to find her standing on top of her counter pulling cooking pots down from the top shelves. She told me she was running out of pots for beans. I offered to help her down so we could wash the ones on her counter. As I reached for a pot, she practically shrieked at me not to lift the lid. Too late. OMG!!! It looked like a fuzzy pink sweater (Pink!!??) had been stuffed into the pot – and the SMELL. We decided not to wash any pots (sorry). Did you know she keeps a black box with SAL scratched on it in the refrigerator? It's your FATHER???!! She said he liked it cold. I didn't know how to respond...

"*I THINK I'M MAD AT YOU, BUT I CAN'T REMEMBER WHAT FOR.*"

Then, as if I needed another universal nudge to do something, my phone rang one evening as Robert and I were settling onto his couch to watch a movie. We'd spent a dirty day clearing brush in his yard and had just finished dinner and a hot shower. I didn't recognize the number on my screen, but I was getting accustomed to random "Fay Calls" and knew I should answer. I was greeted by a woman saying, *"Hello, Carolyn? My name is Sharon. You don't know me, but I'm your mother's neighbor in the back. I don't mean to be nosy, but I just wanted to make sure you knew that there's a man in her backyard. He's pitched a tent and is camping out."*

Robert was already out of his seat and grabbing for his keys as I hurried her off the phone to block him at the door. He was so worked up over the news of some vagrant in my mother's backyard that I didn't trust him to stay cool once he got there. Visions of him speeding into town and physically removing this man and his tent flashed through my mind, closely followed by a jail cell and the morgue. It took a few minutes and some raised voices, but we finally agreed that we needed to stay calm and investigate the scene before we stormed in.

So instead, I called Jeff and Ginny. Our constantly calm Jeff agreed to meet me at Mom's back fence to assess the situation before we decided how to handle things. We all agreed that I'd call Robert if things got out of hand. My goal was to remove this unknown man without a confrontation that my mother might hear, possibly upsetting and frightening her to a point where she wouldn't feel safe there by herself.

I arrived at the back fence where Jeff and Mom's neighbor, Sharon, were already waiting. Smack in the middle of her yard was the tent she'd described, along with a backpack, a worn pair of hiking boots, and a bicycle leaning against the tree. I scanned the yard for any sign of the intruder, but it seemed deserted. Just then I caught some movement in my mother's kitchen window. A man was seated at her table, and it was plain to see that she most certainly wasn't frightened.

We watched from crouched positions while Mom moved around her kitchen, a pot of beans in hand, ladling two scoops into her very skinny guest's bowl. We couldn't hear what they were saying, but just then he threw his head back and laughed. Things appeared harmless, but the reality was there was a stranger in my elderly-mother-who-has-dementia's kitchen, eating potentially lethal beans, depending on which pot she'd reheated from the collection on her counter. I had to do something, but I didn't want anything to escalate into an altercation, especially with him inside her house.

We needed to get him outside where we'd be out of Mom's hearing. My decision was made for me within minutes though, and before we had a chance to devise a plan, he came out the back door and ambled over to his tent. As he began fluffing his sleeping bag and settling in for the night, I took a deep breath and made my move.

"Hello over there! I'm Carolyn, Fay's daughter. Would you mind coming over to the fence so we can chat out of my mother's earshot? What are you doing in my mother's backyard?"

And that's when things escalated into an altercation.

He tossed his pillow back into the tent and took a few steps in our direction. *"I'm spending the night here as your mother's guest,"* he said, obviously not intending to expand on that.

"Well," I replied, "*you can see that my mother has dementia. What'll probably happen tonight is she'll wake up and see you out her window and she won't remember that you're her 'guest.' I can't risk her becoming upset like that. How about we put your tent in the bed of my truck and I drive you down to the fairgrounds where you can camp for free. They even have bathrooms.*"

He looked at me and smiled, "*No, I don't think so. Your mother seems fine to me, and she told me I could stay a week if I wanted.*"

And before I could formulate my response, "constantly calm Jeff" launched himself over the backyard fence and went chest-to-chest with our guest camper, the two of them like Sumo wrestlers inside an imaginary ring, circling and grunting obscenities at each other. I realized quickly that I would've had better luck bringing Robert, who would've swiftly and *quietly* picked him up and removed him. But Jeff and this guy were going at it, and they were getting *louder*. It was no surprise that my mother came out onto her back porch to investigate the noise. She took in the scene and began screeching, "*Leave him alone! He's my friend!*" Add to that the sound of sirens responding to another neighbor's 911 call, and you've got yourselves a genuine redneck party out back on a Saturday night.

Some might feel sorry for the guy, and some might think he was a potentially dangerous, belligerent drifter. I felt both things. I flip-flopped between anger that he'd forced my hand to kick him out and guilt for ruining his lovely evening with my mother.

Hearing my mother plead with them to stop, with that anguished look on her face, was truly heartbreaking. Was I right to interfere? Or had I just needlessly turned a pleasant evening into a disaster. Just then, she spotted me hanging back by the fence and our eyes locked, "*YOU! YOU DID THIS! HOW*

COULD YOU? I WILL NEVER SPEAK TO YOU AGAIN!" Sharon squeezed through the gate and ran over to stand with her while I slinked over to my truck and tried to disappear into the darkness.

When the police arrived, my mother's backyard guest refused to give them his identification and told them it was his right as an American citizen under the United States Constitution to withhold his name from them.

"Is that so?"

With that, they ushered my mother back inside and asked me to leave, promising they'd follow up with me in the morning.

True to their word, I received a call from the sheriff's office early the next day. They informed me that my mother had met her camping guest at the gas station up the street (her new favorite place to shop for milk and ketchup flavored potato chips) and they struck up a conversation. He told her he was bicycling cross-country and camping along the way, so she invited him to camp in her backyard. Simple as that, and it would probably happen again with the next nice man she met. Turns out this gentleman had a warrant for his arrest, tried to run during their questioning, and was the newest resident in our county jail.

Later that morning I nervously drove to her house, scared to death over what she was going to remember from the night before. The doughnuts I brought were a weak peace offering, but I was fresh out of ideas how to handle this. My stomach was in my throat as I got to the front door, and she opened it before I had a chance to knock. She just stood there, not moving to the side, and I braced myself.

Instead, she accepted the bakery box I held up to her and invited me in for coffee. As I followed her into the kitchen, she turned to me and said, *"I think I'm mad at you, but I can't remember what for."* My lungs exploded the breath I'd been holding, and I ruffled her hair (did I mention my mother wasn't a hugger?). *"Nah! There's nothing for you to be mad at, MeeMaw!"* I grinned. And we had a nice cup of coffee with two doughnuts each.

I could finally say I was ready to make some changes to Mom's care and stop hoping for the best, but what were my options, really? Her mobility hadn't deteriorated and she still walked anywhere she wanted, so how could I move her into a care facility and keep her from walking out? She perceived any in-home healthcare visits as a threat. Hell, I was lucky she let me in half the time. And moving anything or cleaning it was out of the question, so my problems were no less monumental than when she'd first arrived.

None of this felt right, regardless of the many conversations I had supporting a move for my mom. My AA group suggested I create a list to read out loud every time I waivered in my resolve. I checked more dementia books out of the library. I even put off calling my brother and sister, fearing they would object. Their disapproval would've paralyzed me even though I knew they weren't going to fly to Idaho to stop me.

I pictured how disloyal I looked, suggesting we move our mother out of her new home and into an institution so soon after we'd placed her in my care. Would they understand the extent to which each new Fay escapade threatened her safety? Or would they just think I'd given up too easily? My track record for controlling her was so poor at this point that I had predictably little confidence in most decisions I made for this moving target I called Mom.

But they didn't object or criticize. They listened to my latest Fay stories as I nervously segued into my decision to move our mother into an assisted living facility. I finished, took a breath, and waited. Each gave me their sympathies, expounded on the enormity of our mother's situation, and gave me the go-ahead to handle things however I chose.

I was relieved, to be sure, but I was also profoundly sad. What else was I hoping for, really? Did I ask them to fly out to help me? No. But they didn't offer, either. The decision was made, and I was capable of implementing it without them, but I'd never felt more alone.

I'd become accustomed to fielding random questions about my brother and sister. *"Where were they?" "Did they fly out to see our mother?" "Were they calling to check in on her?" "Were they calling to check in on me?"* People asked me from time to time about their involvement and whether they helped me, usually after a particularly terrible time I'd had with her. The short answer was no, not really. There were random calls to my mother, usually about the weather, most lasting maybe five minutes.

To be fair, it was next to impossible to have a phone conversation with her. She couldn't carry on two-way communication anymore, just her repeating loop of *"Where are you?" "I want to go home." "When are you coming to get me?" "Are my neighbors stealing my blueberries?" "Your sister keeps me locked here in this house."*

This effectively scared the crap out of Roxanne and Dale. And why wouldn't it? The last time they saw their mother was when she was only mildly forgetful and much slower to anger. This new version was unpredictable and incredibly intimidating. They hadn't experienced the indoctrination I had, and they never quite believed me when I told them they could answer her questions any way they liked because she'd forget within minutes.

I learned early on in my AA meetings that the responsibility of caring for a parent with dementia almost always lands on just one child, even when there are several in the family. It's impossible to predict and often a surprise as to which child shoulders the burden, and it's almost always a source of contention and resentment on the part of that child.

Knowing this was a common family dynamic relieved my conscience. It was almost as if I'd been given permission to feel something uncomfortable and ugly, and still be a good person. I knew the fear they felt, and I equally understood their hesitation to fully involve themselves in Mom's frightening new behaviors. I didn't recognize her anymore and neither did they. I was the one who made the decision to go down and snatch her out of her home, and they were perfectly content in the fact that *Carolyn was handling everything.* But still...

To: Roxanne
From: Carolyn

Hey sis. Are you getting my email updates? Just checking. When you can, let me know that you're getting them. I know you called Mom on Sunday, she told me. Thanks for that. How is she with you on the phone? Don't be scared of the things she says. Just change the subject with anything you think of at the moment. Please keep calling her. It makes her happy. It may not stay with her for long, but I think it's a nice addition to her day and sometimes she remembers it. She's definitely progressing in this thing. Much more forgetful and easily confused. Very paranoid, unfortunately. When you talk to Dale, can you try to get him to call more often?

To: Carolyn
From: Roxanne

Yes, I'm getting your updates, thanks. I call, but she really doesn't stay on the phone for more than 5 or 10 minutes. I told her I was making cookies last Sunday to let the grand kids frost but she didn't care and said she had to go.

To: Roxanne
From: Carolyn

That's just how she is now. Keep calling her. Tell Dale.

SERENITY. IN A HOME.

It was October 2012. Not even six months since I'd set my mother up in her perfect little house on Madison Street. How had it come to this? With a renewed sense of conviction, I began researching senior living places close by. There were only two in my town, The Community Resting Place (TCRP) and Serenity Home. Both were listed as assisted living facilities. I decided quickly that I wanted my mother to live at TCRP. Their resident population was three times as high as Serenity Home, giving her more opportunities to make friends. It was also owned and operated by the county, which I likened to being more professionally managed. In truth, I had no idea whether that was fact, but I was grasping at straws and needed to narrow two establishments down to one.

Several people at my AA meetings had conflicting views on both facilities, which didn't help relieve my anxiety over making the right decision. It seemed like most opinions were based on the quality of staff working there at their given time. This inconsistent subjectivity further undermined my confidence. How was I supposed to choose between the two if I couldn't predict the staffing population?

With my very unscientific choice now made, I called TCRP and was put right through to the intake coordinator. She was so welcoming and understanding as I told her my reason for calling, that within minutes I was giving her *all* my reasons. I felt like I finally had a professional ear to hear my plight, and I didn't hold anything back.

By the end of our conversation (maybe even before that),

I had effectively alarmed the intake coordinator enough for her to inform me they weren't equipped to handle "a problem senior" and that she wished me well.

I was stunned. I hung up with her, crushed and full of regret over having been so forthright. I'd just ruined my chance to move Mom to TCRP, and I wanted a do-over! Would I have lied to her instead? At that point I think my answer would've been, *"Most certainly, yes."* I'd so desperately wanted them to accept her, and I would've said just about anything to make it happen.

Looking back, she wouldn't have lasted a month before being issued an eviction notice for any number of infractions. And where would that have left me? Or her? But this was my first experience with intake interviews, and I hadn't considered that in order to provide the best care for my mother, I had to assess the best fit.

Remember that saying about one door closing and another opening? I found myself facing that second door more times than I imagined possible since taking on Fay. And better outcomes were often achieved than if I'd been allowed to charge right through door number one.

Serenity Home had suddenly become that second door *and* my last option. It was much smaller, privately owned, and I'd heard more mixed opinions about it than I had for TCRP. It consisted of two modest houses: House One was for those needing extra help with daily needs and a quieter environment, and House Two was for the more active residents who could dress themselves and bathe with little assistance.

I called Serenity Home that same afternoon. With carefully chosen words this time, I described my mother and the amount of care I thought she required. The administrator at Serenity Home said, *"Bring her! We can handle her! Let's schedule a tour for you to come see the place."* It really was music to my pretty desperate ears.

We met after their lunch hour the next day for my introductory tour of both houses. House One straight-up scared me. It was dark inside with a hushed atmosphere. Everyone was either in their bed or tipping sideways in a chair out in the main area, fast asleep. I told myself it didn't matter. Fay wouldn't be living in that house. House Two seemed more like someone's personal home with a large sedentary "family" seated in the living room with the TV blaring.

I couldn't help but be disappointed. It didn't compare well with The Community Resting Place, with its planned activities and a more active population with whom my mother could've interacted. TCRP even had a van that carted them into town every Tuesday; my mom would've loved that.

I left my tour of Serenity Home feeling unsettled. *I wanted so badly to like it.* I'd hoped to allay my misgivings toward House One after seeing the more active House Two, but that didn't happen, either.

I chided myself for being too exacting. I'd made myself a promise to watch over her and guard her, and I reasoned that I could do that much better with her close by. And Serenity Home was my only local choice. If I'm being honest, I'd already decided to move my mother there after my rejection from TCRP. So despite my reservations, I returned the following day to sign the paperwork necessary to reserve a room for her.

It was time to begin laying the groundwork for the move by playing on Mom's never ending loop, *"When is Dale coming to get me and bring me home?"* I decided to turn it into the reason for her move.

"Dale is putting in for his vacation time at work (he still hadn't found a job) *and then he's going to drive here* (and his driver's license was still revoked) *and move you back home* (that house we just packed you out of and sold)... *But first we need to move you to a temporary place because we're going to*

box up all your things for the moving van, and you won't have
a bed to sleep in or pots and pans to cook with."

I had to repeat that story to her dozens of times. It was one
of the few things she didn't question, and it always settled her.

> **To:** Carolyn
> **From:** Jolle
>
> It sounds like you're making progress toward getting
> your mother moved to a **safer environment.** I know this
> is a very difficult time, and we can only hope that she
> adjusts well to the care facility. Please don't feel guilty
> about what you're doing. It is the best for your mom
> even if she doesn't understand that. You are doing the
> only thing possible under the circumstances. I look
> forward to seeing you at the next meeting. Take care of
> **yourself.**

So with the help of family, ex-family, and friends, I
launched another plan. And it started with Sam. My mother
always liked him. She was raised in a time when the man was
the head of the household, and Sam exuded authority. It
connected nicely with my mother's mindset, and it came in
handy during our maneuverings.

The plan was for Ginny and Jeff to take Fay apple picking
at Sam's while Robert and I packed up her two dressers and a
few of her personal things, purchased a twin mattress set at
Beck's Furniture, and hauled everything to her new room at
Serenity Home.

After apples, Jeff, Ginny, and my mother would come to
Serenity Home to have lunch in the dining room and then
they'd introduce her to her new room.

> **To:** Ginny, Jeff, Sam
> **From:** Carolyn
>
> We should keep everything as simple as possible.
> Script:
> 1. Fay wants to go home, so Carolyn is making it happen.
> 2. Carolyn will ride along in the moving truck to make sure
>   all her things are safe.

3. It takes 3 weeks (1 to get there, 1 to unload, and 1 to drive back).
4. Dale is asking for vacation time at work and will drive out sometime after that to get her.
5. Meanwhile, she needs a short-term place with a kitchen because her house will be empty, and she can't stay there without furniture. (What if she demands to go by her house so she can confirm it's empty??!!)

*** We need to start using Dale's name as often as possible from now on. This way the focus will be off me. *** AM I THE ONLY ONE WHO IS TERRIFIED???

Ginny, thanks for setting her hair. She didn't remember where her curlers were? Wow. No, she never used a blow dryer. She's dry within an hour. And yes, she loves Shirley Temple.

To: Carolyn
From: Ginny

I'm heading over now with some packing tape. If it's any comfort, I can understand Fay's agitation. The moving boxes remind her something's up, but she can't remember what it is. It might be helpful to keep giving her the simple outline of what to expect, or even write it down on a calendar or note paper.

Hang in there, Carolyn, and keep remembering that you have us behind you.

Robert and I spent the morning setting up her new room with her bed, her dressers, and as many of her personal favorites as we could fit. Then, right before lunchtime we skedaddled. While Mom was great with Jeff and Ginny, she was less so with us, and if she was going to act out in front of anyone, it would be me.

Jeff and Ginny had spent a lovely morning at the farm with Mom and Sam and were in good spirits, at least hopeful ones, as they pulled up to Serenity Home. I don't know if it was the look of the courtyard that gave it away, or the "Welcome to Serenity Home" sign at the driveway entrance, but some alarm fired off in Mom's brain when they parked the car and got out. Ginny opened my mother's door and leaned in to help her out, but Fay wouldn't budge from her seat. She sat there staring straight ahead, and every time they tried to coax her out, she shook her head, repeating, *"No! No! No! No! No!"* until it turned into a shriek, and they knew they were in over their heads.

Instead of calling me, they called Sam. Their reasoning was that he'd just spent the morning with my mother, and they'd had a good visit. And he *had* offered his help if they needed it, saying he was just five minutes away. Five minutes later, Sam walked over to their car, opened the passenger side door, and squatted down, *"C'mon Fay, let's go have some lunch."* She didn't even hesitate as she took his hand while everyone collectively exhaled. They went inside to enjoy lasagna, salad, and garlic rolls. No, they didn't call her daughter for help – they called her daughter's ex-husband – and yeah, when they told me the story it may have stung for seven seconds. Truth is, I was incredibly relieved that was what they did.

Sam ended up staying with Mom for the rest of the afternoon while Jeff and Ginny went home. He didn't suggest a walk, fearing Mom would refuse to go back inside her new home afterward. After a light evening meal of sandwiches and fruit cups, Mom decided to take a nap and even let Sam help her lie down and tuck her in. Ginny called me afterward to fill me in, and thus began my daily updates while we were in the agreed upon *"seven day cooling off period"* recommended by the Serenity Home administrator for me to stay away and let her settle in.

They told me it was their experience that sometimes a newly admitted resident needed a week or so to acclimate to their new surroundings and maybe divert a little anger away from the family member who put them there. It was agreed that Denise and Ginny would stop by every day and report back to me. I don't think I can truly convey just how tough it was for me to stay away that week, but it was without a doubt the wisest suggestion they made.

Mom was *mad,* like the stomping around, refusing to eat, talking trash about me kind of mad. Every photo of me she had was torn up and thrown into the garbage can. She told the staff stories about me that I prayed they'd have the experience to know the difference between truth and fabrication. I was a constant source of suspicion and the general topic all day, for seven days. And then it was time for me to make my first visit.

I called Serenity Home on the seventh day to see what time I should drop by and was told the administrator wanted to speak with me and would call me right back. Um, okay... I received her call about an hour later and it went something like, *"Hi Carolyn, it's everyone's opinion here that your mother isn't quite ready to receive you yet. We think you should give it another week."* I stood there blinking. You would think I'd be relieved not to have to subject myself to who knows what she'd be serving up. But I wasn't.

The ache I felt in my gut was indescribable – I so utterly needed to see my mother that it consumed me. I fretted about her all day and slept very little that entire second week. I wasn't just missing her; I was feeling this incredible amount of regret that I'd put her in this place against her will and removed any small amount of independence she'd had. I'd stripped away her freedom to take her walks whenever she wanted, her pots of beans, even her endlessly brewed carafes of coffee. And now I couldn't even be there to help her transition into her new home. Of course, that was the whole point – *she didn't want me there to help her transition.*

A second week went by, and I received the same recommendation when I called – to wait yet another week. I was beside myself with worry, impatience, and tremendous remorse.

Denise, Ginny, and Sam were faithfully visiting Mom and sending me updates that she was doing fine. They would gently answer each of my questions regarding her attitude towards me, which were always tagged with, *"and you know she doesn't mean it... it's just the disease."*

To: Carolyn
From: Denise

Your mom was in rare form today. She was sharing peanut butter and crackers with all the residents in the living room, moving from one to the next with her full plate. I hesitate to tell you that every single photo of you is in shreds. It looks like one of the caregivers fished them out of her trash can and tried taping them back together. There are about a half dozen that have been pieced together on her dresser. And guess who's sharing her bed with her? Yep! SAL in his shiny black box. She pulled back the covers just to show me her secret. I think he comforts her.

Week three was over and I was finally given the green light to try a visit with her. We decided Ginny would arrive ahead of me and I would casually drop in, which was another good plan. Mom raised her three children to be polite and socially correct. It was a relief to see that she still followed her own rules of etiquette when another person was present.

I hadn't seen my mother in 21 days. I pulled into the parking lot and sat there, sweating that nervous sweat you get under your armpits before public speaking or some other dreaded event. *"This is so stupid,"* I thought. But I can't convey to you how petrified I was to go inside. Visions of my mother screaming at me to *"Get Out! How could you do this to me?!"* flooded my brain. Or worse, tears and declarations of how scared and helpless she felt, all alone and wanting to go home. Having Ginny there gave me some reassurance and a sense of protection. And we were depending on her calm presence to keep Mom from tearing into me.

I entered through the front door of the main living area where two caregivers were waiting for me with solemn faces. They said nothing, just pointed toward her room down the hall.

When she saw me come into her room, she got a snide, twisted look on her face and turned away from me. I hadn't expected that. I was sure she was going to run down the list of my bad daughter traits, loud enough for the whole house to hear. Instead, she refused to acknowledge me. She didn't look at me; she didn't say a word. I tried to engage her. I asked her direct questions, but she continued to ignore me, staring at the bathroom door.

The silent pauses were deafening and painful. I tried to make small talk with Ginny, hoping Mom would become interested in our conversation and join in, but it was so one sided and awkward that after several attempts Ginny signaled me that I should leave. I stayed for about 15 minutes more and then said my goodbyes to Ginny and to the side of my mother's face.

The hallway leading from my mother's room to the main living area felt endless as I made my exit, trying to shake off the ringing in my ears. I remember holding it together just long enough to walk through the house and out to my truck. My keys fell out of my purse and as I stooped to pick them up, I released a sob so strangled that I vomited on my shoes. No one came out of the house to see about it, but I was quite sure they were standing just inside the windows, watching.

I find it incredible now, looking back, how profoundly my mother's behavior affected not only me, but everyone around her. None of us knew how to treat her. She was human like anyone else, but she was emotionally powerful and downright scary when she was unhappy. She didn't raise her voice, she didn't use profanity, but she had this way of showing her displeasure that was unnerving. We were all afraid of her, even the caregivers, I think.

I went back every day for the first couple of weeks and I guess you could say things eventually settled down. I would bring a little present each time I visited, like a gorgeous ripe pear or a jumbo cookie from the bakery – things I thought might get a reaction from her. At first she wouldn't acknowledge my gifts, but then I'd receive a report from Denise or Ginny that she'd eaten the pear I'd left or offered them a bite of the cookie *"that my daughter brought by."*

Denise and Ginny tag teamed drop ins. So among the three of us, Mom had a visitor every day, and sometimes two. The caregivers reported minimal mischief from her. No serious escape attempts, she followed directions readily – just like she taught her daughter – and was their idea of a nicely transitioned resident. It hadn't quite been two months, and she'd already forgotten why she was mad at me.

Whenever I arrived, she'd light up with a big smile, then she'd scowl and say, *"I know I'm mad at you for something..."* I'd just laugh and tell her I was sure it was nothing.

$\mathcal{M}$ONDAY, MONDAY...
AND ALL THE DAYS IN BETWEEN

Year Two – Stage 3
(Mild Cognitive Impairment)

Spring returned to North Idaho, and one day I pulled up to see that the maintenance man had tilled my mother a small space near the side of the house for a flower garden, which Ginny helped her turn into a vegetable plot, since *"flowers were a waste of good garden space."* My job was to bring by any kind of vegetable seed Mom would like to grow, which meant every kind. That 8x10 plot nearly burst with every sort of vegetable we could squeeze into its neat rows.

It thrilled her to witness her first sprouts break through the soil. She became so fixated on them that she would water those tiny green shoots to the point of drowning. She spent each morning walking the perimeter, hands behind her back and stooped over as she peered down each row for signs of activity. Survivors were rewarded with a healthy glug of water. Then she'd retrace her steps to the hose bib to refill her emptied watering jug and lug it back to the garden, sloshing water all over her pant legs, and begin again.

Fay became a garden fixture, patrolling rows and traipsing to the hose bib, pausing only long enough to join the others when they called her in for meals.

Within days, that garden was too muddy to enter, and in an effort to save it (and the carpets), the caregivers were instructed to hide the jug, which Fay managed to locate within one day; and finally, to shut the water supply off to the outside hose bib. She would've been furious if she hadn't been so utterly confused by it.

Not easily defeated, my determined mother could be seen making trips back and forth to the side of the house, where she'd crank on the bib handle and wait. When no water came out, she'd lower herself down onto her knees and peer up into the faucet to see what went wrong. They told me she did this dozens of times while they watched from a window, keeping out of her line of sight. She changed her strategy and began hanging out near the hose bib, busying herself by pulling weeds and then randomly reaching over to turn the handle.

It only took my resourceful mother another half day to come up with Plan C, and she'd now become a steady source of entertainment for the residents in House Two. Everyone pretended not to notice, snickering as she stealthily entered and exited her bedroom, Dixie cup in hand. Shared laughter would erupt from the living room as she shuffled out the front door, trying not to jostle her full cup of water to feed her half-drowned darlings. It was better than any TV game show they had on during the achingly long hours of the day, and Fay was too focused to notice.

She never tried to explain her soaked shirt or the water down the front of her pants, and no one mentioned them. And several weeks later, those tough little plants produced strawberries, string beans, and tomatoes for her to harvest.

Mom's garden kept her occupied all summer. Combined with her daily walks with Ginny or Denise, regular mealtime breaks, and a couple visits from me each week, and she was a busy girl. She'd almost become a pleasure to be with, or at least more manageable. The trepidation I'd felt during my first visits after her cooling down period seemed like a vague memory, and my biggest challenge now was to fill our time with fun, harmless activities that didn't send her down the rabbit hole. I brought magazines, small puzzles, and nail polish. Sometimes I'd even bring a sewing kit and ask her to help me replace a button or fix a tear.

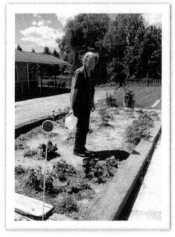

~ All that work...
and all her attention ~

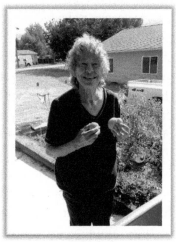

~ I think she
carried them all day ~

Our walks, though, had stopped after only the first few. The last one ended with her darting to the parking lot and demanding to know which car was mine. (Oh dear...) I didn't have the quick wit to tell her I'd walked there (that would've been brilliant), so I pointed to my truck. She strode quickly to the side of it, lifted the handle (thank God I'd locked it), and turned on me, *"Come on, let's go! I want you to take me home NOW. Call Dale. I want him to come get me. Let's go! I'm not going back inside there."*

My mother's pleas to take her away from the very situation I had put her in felt like a knife slicing into my ribs. No amount of practice had prepared me for a quick, reassuring response and the lava-hot river that flowed through my chest threatened to spew out of my mouth. Nothing was the same with me and my mother as it was with Ginny or Denise, or anyone else for that matter. She never threatened them with refusing to go back inside, and she never pleaded with them to take her away.

To: Denise
From: Carolyn

Mom's pension check came in the mail today, but should I bring it to her? She hasn't asked about it since we moved her to Serenity Home. Maybe she's finally forgotten about it. If I give it to her, will I be setting myself up for misery each month again?

BTW, I'm taking her to Kaniksu Health for her appointment today, 2pm. It's to renew her diabetes meds and to complete the entrance form for Serenity Home. (They're going to administer something called a "general mental state" test – or something like that for dementia). Think I'll wait out in the lobby...

To: Carolyn
From: Denise

Ha! Ha! The lobby sounds like a smart idea. I'll see if she remembers anything about her pension check tomorrow when we walk. She hasn't mentioned your thieving ways in a while. You might be right that she's forgotten about it.

Denise's walks with Mom were so different than mine had been. Mom behaved, for one thing. I was always one part jealous to two parts relieved when she reported back that they'd had fun on their walks. "Fun" hadn't been a word in my Fay-vocabulary for a couple of years. Denise would arrive promptly each morning after the gym and ready to walk. Mom would also be ready and seated at the front door, her coat buttoned to her neck and her hat in her lap. Sometimes she'd be wearing two pairs of pants, no clue why, and no amount of convincing could get her to remove one.

Off they'd go, Mom with her hat screwed down onto her head, excited for their neighborhood escapade of the day. Sometimes they collected pretty rocks along the road, or they'd bribe the neighbor's dog with biscuits to keep him from rushing them at the fence. But Mom's all-time favorite was scavenging all the gorgeous fruit trees in everyone's yards – fronts, sides, and backs – that they passed.

Denise would hurry to the front door to ask if it was okay for them to pick something, but Mom was already picking by the time her knock was answered. The owners of the trees would wave to them from their porches and tell Mom she could come back as often as she wanted – big mistake. Fay may not have remembered her way back home, but she never forgot where the fruit trees were or that particular owner's promise, and it was all Denise could do to carry their load back to the house after their walks.

And consider, this was every walk. Every day. That's a lot of fruit.

With an abundance of fruit comes fruit flies, so I wasn't surprised to receive a call from Serenity Home about the swarming pests and foul odor of rotting fruit coming from Fay's room. They'd tried every remedy to confiscate the hoarded bounty packed into her drawers, from diverting her attention to sneaking into her room when she was showering, but *she had a photographic memory when it came to what belonged to her,* and she was currently throwing a fit about her stolen fruit.

Ginny was the mastermind who came up with a solution that satisfied everybody, *"Let's can fruit!"* Staff opened the kitchen for them and thus began the not-quite-sweet-enough, sometimes runny jars of any kind of fruit spread you could imagine, depending on the harvest.

To: Carolyn
From: Ginny

Your Mom was in prime form today, happy as can be picking fruit. First it was the plum tree where we picked two bagsful, stowing them to go back to retrieve. Then we met several people on our walk, with friendly Fay asking folks ever-so-politely if we could harvest their windfall fruit. I think we met three separate neighbors today, and made off with gifted apples, plums, and tomatoes – the latter given to us by a suspender-wearing older guy named "Ben" who reminded me of Sal. THEN we hit the mother lode – elderberry trees down by the hospital! Fay was ecstatic, humming (she does that, doesn't she!?) and busily filling her plastic bags as full as could be. It pained her to leave any on the tree, but the trees were full, and we only had two spare bags.

On the trip home, walking uphill with our fingers being gouged by the bag handles from the weight of the berries, Fay exclaimed: "I wouldn't want to live *any other place!*" When we got back to Serenity Home, we showed off our good fortune and started the tedious job of separating berry from stem. When I left, we had half a *huge* metal bowl full already, and Fay was still humming. I plan to do some jam making with her, maybe Tuesday.

As happy as this made me, I'd learned that with every solution we found, my mother's dementia had the uncanny ability to create new and different sets of problems. This time was no different. Ginny's canning project with Mom quickly turned into a daily fight between staff and Mom in the kitchen. My mother loved being in the kitchen and now that she was back in one, she couldn't understand why she was being blocked from regular entry. Serenity Home's policy was that no resident was allowed unattended in the kitchen for safety reasons, so the lower door was kept locked and the lights turned off. This infuriated her.

She'd walk by that kitchen door twenty times a day and grab hold of the doorknob to see if it would give. And sometimes it did – an unfortunate slip-of-mind by a random caregiver who'd forgotten about Fay – and that's when she'd go to work, opening each cabinet door to see what was inside. I can only imagine the sight of all those gaping cabinets for the next unsuspecting caregiver who wandered into the kitchen afterward.

I got the call from the administrator within a week that we had a serious problem. My mother's insistence to be in the kitchen was in direct conflict with their safety requirements from the state. And this constant back-and-forth kitchen door duel between Mom and the staff was upsetting the entire house, *and* they were looking to me for a remedy.

My mother hadn't been there a year yet and this was the fourth problem call I'd received. Each one was a new tennis ball whizzing past my head, but we'd figured them out together up until now. How was I going to solve this new problem when *they* didn't have a solution either! I was scared to death the next call from them was going to be the one stating she was more trouble than they'd imagined, and they couldn't continue to keep her. There was no other place for her to go. I'd burned my bridge with The Community Resting Place after telling them the truth about her behavior, and she certainly couldn't go back to living on her own. I was desperate for some way around this.

And I was stumped. How was I going to keep Mom out of their kitchen when I couldn't possibly be there each time the infraction occurred? There was no way to monitor who remembered to lock the kitchen door and who forgot. And my mother was impossible to reason with, so there was that.

The first thing I did was ramp up my visits. I figured since Denise was out walking with her every morning after the gym, I'd use that time to hurry home, grab a quick breakfast and a shower. I could be pulling into the driveway just as Denise was leaving. That would put me right in front of lunch time. If I could keep Mom occupied and away from the kitchen door (and the tempting sounds of clinking and clattering dishes), maybe she'd forget about her kitchen fixation.

She didn't forget, though. Like reminding a toddler not to touch that (insert your favorite thing here), she went back to the door every few minutes, and I'd start all over again with some new diversion. Nothing I tried was working, and by Day Three I was already defeated. I knew I couldn't keep this new schedule going, and we were no closer to a solution.

The weekday caregiver had begun letting us set the table for her, which quickly turned into table clearing, wipe down, and sweeping. With her new list of duties, Mom was too busy to worry about what wonders awaited her behind the kitchen door. I was thrilled, and the caregiver was ecstatic, but for different reasons. She'd confided in me that she hated getting lunches ready for the residents. She complained about the menu, the lack of available ingredients in the pantry, and the work involved – especially the cleanup.

Aha! I'd found my solution to the kitchen door duels and our rabbit hole dives! I called the administrator and presented *"Monday Lunch Days with Fay and Carolyn."* I offered to shop, chop, prepare and serve one meal every week, with my mother's assistance, of course. I even threw in that we'd clean up afterward. I suggested that maybe if Mom had some supervised time in the kitchen, it wouldn't feel so off limits (and so tempting), and I'd be there with her, giving the Monday caregiver a break from lunches and cleanup. My additional offer to pay for the ingredients sealed our deal, and Monday Lunch Days with Fay and Carolyn began.

Mom was overjoyed! She had no idea she was being supervised or limited in any way. The kitchen door was being opened and the lights turned on to behold an enormous, magical kitchen containing every size pot, pan, and mixing bowl she could imagine. And that was her reality for the next two hours. The Monday caregiver was equally thrilled to have a break from kitchen duties, as was the administrator, having one less group meal to purchase every week.

We prepped, served, and cleaned our way through our Mondays, and they quickly became everyone's favorite lunch day. I'd dress Mom in a frilly apron or party hat, if she let me, and I always made a big presentation to her of all the beautiful ingredients I'd hauled in as I removed them from the box and placed them onto the kitchen counter for her to inspect. She never seemed to notice that everything was already chopped and portioned out. She was happy enough to oversee carefully placing everything into the baking dish before inserting it into the waiting oven.

I compiled a list of interesting casseroles that would satisfy a large group of aging adults with a variety of health restrictions, personal tastes, and number of teeth. It wasn't easy. Desserts were a breeze as long as pudding, cake, or ice cream was involved. And I took requests. I even named them. We had Cheesy Cheeks Casserole, Busty Betty Broccoli Bake, and my favorite, Slutty Sausage and Spinach. That one became the most requested from the male residents – go figure. Everyone would be seated, and then Mom and I would remove the pan from the oven and parade it around the table. We had a rule that everyone had to *"oooh!"* and *"ahhh!"* before I agreed to serve it up. It was our thing.

Fay was in her element on Monday lunch days. She set the tables, poured the waters, and helped me pass the plates. She even loved to clean up. I'd wash while she dried, although most things were placed in the dishwasher, which was difficult to explain to my very conventional mother who was convinced we could do a better job by hand.

Our Mondays together became the balm we needed to navigate this new mother-daughter dynamic we'd found ourselves in. *We had two hours of together-time that was focused on a project,* distracting her from her loop of nasty comments about my clothes, makeup, and lack of morality for stealing from my own mother. Even her constant barrage of *"When am I going home?"* questions were quelled that day. Well, for the most part they were.

To: Ginny
From: Carolyn

It was a bad day in Fayland today. I'm hesitant to tell it
– you might stop liking her. She tested every bit of my
patience... Kathy taking on the whole team in their work
truck, staff stealing from her at night, Rose peeing in her
pants and needing diapers – and isn't that SO funny,
the nurse's big ass (yep, she said ass), staff stealing
food from the kitchen and taking it home, and here's a
new one: Dale DID INDEED come to fetch her, and he
didn't get lost....I TOLD HIM TO GO HOME instead and
am keeping her here against her will, AND I have the
nerve to only come see her on Mondays because I'm
just SOOO BUSY (insert twisted face here). Then there
was, "What are you doing with my check? Where is it?
What bank? I don't have a bank here! YOU closed out
my account!"

I couldn't stand it any longer – all this in one visit! So I
told her that the truck story about Kathy was NOT TRUE
and very ugly. She should never say those things. I told
her it was very sad about Rose needing diapers and
isn't it hard getting old. And to the last question about
banking, I said, "Hey! Do you have any hand lotion? My
hands are so dry from doing the dishes." And off she
went to get some. She came out of her room empty
handed about ten minutes later and asked me what I
was doing there.

And you absolutely did NOT put that lovely pine bark
down – somebody is messing with her garden. And you
absolutely did NOT come help her plant peppers. And
it "sticks in her craw" (never heard her say that word)
that no one helps her and that they just sit there on their
big fat butts and give her orders to weed it so they can
someday eat all her hard work. So I said, "Well then, I
think you should protest and not work another day in
that labor camp! C'mon, let's go tell them right now that
you're not going to step foot in that garden again."

To that, she didn't reply and moved on to "Where's my
coffee cup?"

The BEST part was when she told me she was "sick of
me" because I think I'm so special when everyone
fawns over me like I'm a princess. Then she literally

smacked me on the back six times (hard!) until I took hold of her wrist to stop her while she said, "It's the pats on the back you're after." I responded calmly that it was nice to be thanked once in a while, but that I enjoyed making lunch for everyone so I could spend time with her. Then went out to my truck and cried. Feeling low.

To: Carolyn
From: Ginny

Sorry to hear this – it seems to be getting harder for mostly you. Some daughters and sons eventually choose to stop visits altogether when visits agitate/anger their parents too much. In the least you can set firm limits like you did, which can even include walking out (with an explanation why) when abuse doesn't stop. Not sure how to do this with a casserole in the oven however :)

No need to censor what you tell me. It doesn't make me dislike her because I see it mostly as a projection of her feelings of helplessness. When you take away Fay's invented stories and human targets of her anger, I see someone feeling very confused, powerless, and jealous of what was taken from her by dementia.

When I arrived on Sunday Fay had two Serenity Home garden tools wrapped up tightly in a bag stored in her drawer to give to me. Staff told me about them when I got there, and Fay led me to them first thing because she is now perceiving Serenity Home as stealing from me. I had to tell her that they were Serenity Home's tools, not mine, and Fay returned them quietly to the shed to save face. She is constantly taking things from the kitchen (cookies, etc.), wrapping them and giving them to me secretly to take away. Always conspiring against the "enemy."

I once again convinced Fay to let me curl her hair Sunday, under the same fib about me being in beauty school. Works like a charm. Her hair was looking kind of dirty. I don't envy them trying to get Fay to bathe. I can only imagine it must be a battle of wills. Off to see Fay again soon. *Was* thinking of bringing the rest of the pine bark...

To: Ginny
From: Carolyn

Your response helps. I'll try to remember that her level of nastiness equals her level of confusion. I'm just glad she's nice to you and Denise. Weird, she doesn't ever try to steal things from the kitchen when I'm there. Must be some gift just for you. Then again, she swears you never help her in the garden and she's mad at you. Then you show up and she's ready to go, like it's your routine. Different dynamics with different people, I guess. She's practically slapstick with Denise. Giving each other noogies and punches in the arm. She never does that with you, and certainly not me.
As always, thank you for everything you do. What do I owe you for the pine bark?

I had my hands full keeping Mom busy those days. She was the most active of the dozen residents there and wasn't allowed to venture outside beyond the garden alone, since the caregiver on duty was needed inside the house.

Even with Denise's morning walks, Ginny's visits a few times a week, and my Monday lunches, Fay had a lot of down time.

Staff realized quickly that Mom needed a steady stream of distractions throughout the day just to keep her happy and compliant. They'd started leaving the broom out so she could sweep the floors whenever she wanted and a dust cloth in a basket marked, "Fay." Ingenious! They even brought her the laundry basket of towels to fold, which kept her busy for a while, and we were all granted several weeks of smooth routine.

Now that Fay was secure in her new position as "housekeeper" at Serenity Home, she began pitching in when she deemed help was needed with the other, less mobile residents. She tried to lift Bea when no one was nearby to respond to Bea's requests for help, or she'd pick up a resident's spoon and feed them when the caregiver was giving her attention to someone else.

Seemingly harmless actions in Fay's eyes, but potentially disastrous in staff's, and hence, another *"We have a problem"* call from Serenity Home. We were all in agreement that telling my mother not to do something pretty much guaranteed she would. But rather, distraction had an amazing effect on ending an undesirable action, like feeding another resident or trying to lift Bea.

So Mom became the official laundry folder and was given a daily basketful of clean towels to fold. When done, the caregiver brought the basket to the back room, dumped it out, and would then present Fay with a new basketful of the same towels to fold – press repeat. They could keep this up all day long. When she wasn't sweeping the floor, wiping tables, doing crafts, making lunch, or walking with Denise, she was folding towels. Anything to keep her away from Bea.

To: Ginny
From: Carolyn

Good day today! She helped me deliver every plate to the table and cleared the dishes by herself. She had a thing about the oven today, incessantly checking the status of lunch (Mom! It'll never bake with the oven door open!). She doesn't remember where her puzzles came from. She asked me about her new coat, and when I told her I'd brought it, she snipped, "Then why did you hide it from me in my closet?" She informed me that you now live there and isn't it strange that you used to be her neighbor in Georgia. I handed Mom another roll of cash – ones and fives and tens – when I got there and she stuffed it in her pocket. I asked her where she put it as I was leaving. She said she never got anything from me and insisted she only had her own wad. I told her to look in her other pocket and boy was she surprised to pull out that new roll! Guess I didn't need to bring it after all. She's convinced that Rose is coming into her room when she goes on her walks. The proof is in the two ice cream wrappers she found in her bathroom trash can, obviously left there by Rose. Should I say something to warn staff?

To: Carolyn
From: Ginny

I'd let staff know. Geez, if you were ever doubting your decision to move your mom there...

THE COMMUNITY RESTING PLACE - WE BEGIN AGAIN.

Year Three – Stage 3, some 4
(Mild Cognitive Impairment / Mild Dementia)

Another year passed quickly, and although we watched new residents move into House Two, we watched quite a few more than that leave. My mother had finally stopped asking about her car, and rarely showed me the money she kept in a Ziploc baggie in her pants pocket for the day she planned to break out. She was becoming what I read in my books as "institutionalized." She recognized Serenity Home as her home, she let them lead her through her weekly bathing routine, and at some point they even allowed her to serve herself coffee from the kitchen.

Sounds like a perfectly reasonable time to uproot her and cause chaos again, right? Not right, but that's what I did. While she had adapted to the routine of group home living, and everyone was on board with schemes to keep her busy, her down time behavior was rapidly becoming an increasingly bigger problem.

In a house that small, with just a dozen residents and usually 1.5 caregivers (when you count the floater who bounced between the two houses as needed), negative human nature can rear its ugly head even in the best of circumstances.

I discovered that my mother talked back, and sometimes this was met by an indignant reprimand from the caregiver, which led to hurt feelings and stony silences between the two. I'd observed a few occurrences myself, and when Ginny and

Denise both mentioned a few tiffs they'd witnessed, I knew things were escalating in the wrong direction. The unfortunate scolding, shouting, and general roughness I had seen being directed at some of the other residents had somehow been tolerable for me to ignore, as long as they weren't directed at my mother. And now it appeared as though they were.

To: Carolyn
From: Ginny

Bad weather for a walk today. We sat in the main room and chatted, and Fay was upbeat. Staff however was anything but upbeat, and the yelling and scolding of Bea in the corner chair really got to me. It almost makes me want to be a whistleblower or at least tape record her – I had that horrible gut feeling you get when one has to witness abuse *("BEA!!! I SAID STAY IN YOUR CHAIR!!!! YOU'RE GOING TO FALL! Do you HEAR ME???!!!! BEA!!!!!!")*. I was very conflicted today, with the choice to risk my relationship with staff, or give poor Bea the protection and care she deserves – it really seemed like straight out verbal abuse to me. Then staff went on a (loud) tirade in front of all of us about the other staff not giving Bea enough anxiety medication at the right time, and now SHE has to deal with it. All Bea wanted to do was go lie in her bed because she thought it was nighttime. Yikes. Even Fay said staff had been doing this all day.

But back to Fay. She must've told me six times that "that old Sam came to visit me today and we laughed and laughed." When Jeff came to get me, she went out to the car to see Molly, and then gave Jeff a big kiss on the cheek which took him completely by surprise. She has been so affectionate lately.

To: Ginny
From: Carolyn

It's with mixed feelings that I read this. But that's no fault of yours. I love that Mom had a great day. It's funny how she loves male company. I know she has a warm spot for Sam, which was never the case when we were married – isn't that interesting? Sam told me he'd been there to visit and that he had words with staff after he heard her yelling at one of the residents.

What would you do if your mom lived there? In an ideal world, Hell yes, blow that whistle. And I should be the first and loudest blower since it's my mother we're talking about. But I've ALSO seen how things work over there, and there ARE NO SECRETS. If I say something, it will absolutely get back to staff exactly who said it. And she takes things so personally. All our relationships would be ruined with her. And think of the repercussions with Mom. Would she take it out on her? And are those things reasons enough to NOT say something? Is Bea being abused? Have I touched on the same concerns as yours, or are yours different? Let's compare.

There's something about the nature of needing a thing so badly that you'd do almost anything to avoid losing it, even when you know you should. I NEEDED Serenity Home. In my mind, I had nowhere else to place my mother. I clearly couldn't keep her, I'd single-handedly eliminated The Community Resting Place as an option, and the 70-mile round trip to Sandpoint felt like an eternity. I glanced past every little waving red flag, and much like the frog in the slow-to-boil pot, my alarms hadn't gone off immediately or regularly enough at Serenity Home to move me to action. My complaints were few, actually, and the ones I did have I chalked up to human nature, our town's small caregiver workforce, and a low pay scale. These ladies had a tougher job than I'd ever want to take on, so who was I to judge them when they lost their cool or slacked off occasionally? That was how I rationalized it while my mom lived there, until I couldn't anymore.

Ginny and I decided to each draft a letter and send them a few days apart from each other. They'd *never* figure out that they'd come from us that way, right? Not right, again.

Would I do this again, knowing there'd likely be fallout from the caregiver in question? My short answer is "yes." My longer answer is I'm glad I had another option ready for my mother if shit hit the fan, and I had a hunch it would. What was going on at Serenity House needed to be exposed, for sure, but once it was, I had no guarantee that the bad behavior was going to end. And it certainly could get worse. People are people, and as much as I liked to think I could demand professionalism from the folks there, it wasn't always the case. The only thing in my control was whether Mom stayed or whether I moved her.

The letters were sent, and let's just say that XXXX was taken aside, most likely shown the letters, and absolutely figured out who sent them. The frosty reception I received the next time I visited left no doubt about that. Same with Ginny. Same with Denise, unfortunately. We even left poor Denise out of it, thinking only two letters would keep XXXX uncertain as to which two of the three of us were the culprits. Instead, we were all to blame. I didn't waste any time removing my mother from her current situation and quickly made arrangements to relocate her into the larger, more traditional assisted living home in our town. Yes, I'm referring to The Community Resting Place.

You may remember that I had spoken with the intake manager at TCRP more than a year earlier about my mother, and she had assessed immediately that Fay wasn't a fit at their facility (and she was right). Well, she remembered me right away and she also hadn't forgotten my Fay horror stories. But I was convinced that Mom's year-plus stay at Serenity Home had acclimated her to the world of assisted living and she was vastly different from the problematic senior I had described back then. My challenge was to convince the intake manager.

I described her daily routines, explained that she needed more interaction with more active residents, and that I was worried for her well-being if I left her at Serenity Home. She didn't sound convinced and informed me that we would need to schedule an interview to assess Mom's potential fit with

TCRP before she could consider her admittance.

Well THAT wasn't going to work. There was no doubt in my mind that Fay would totally blow it in a formal interview. I needed to think quickly before I committed my mother to an immediate "fail" before she even had a chance to show them she would do well there. I was getting surprisingly good at navigating Mom's overly active brain, and I could out-fib the best of them by now. I suggested bringing Fay to lunch in their dining room that week so the manager could meet her in a more relaxed environment and assess her that way, *without making her uncomfortable in an official interview.*" She agreed and we set a Thursday date.

Denise and I hatched a new plan, and this time it went beautifully. I dropped in at Serenity Home unannounced on Thursday to pick my mother up for lunch. I didn't want to give them something to wonder about by telling them in advance, especially since I was their *Monday* Girl *and* I never put my mother in my truck.

"Come on, Mom! Let's go have lunch. My treat!" I said as I breezed into the living room where she was watching TV with the others. She bounced out of her recliner without hesitating and skittered to her room for her coat. It made me sad to realize she'd probably go anywhere with anyone rather than sit in that living room with the others, but it reinforced my decision to move her.

The courtyard we entered at TCRP was simply beautiful, with fall mums in bloom and a gurgling water fountain. There were even butterflies flitting around them and my mother was enthralled by every detail. The resident cat was lounging on the pavers in the sun, tail flicking as my mother stooped to stroke it and coo. I couldn't have orchestrated a more inviting scene for her. I opened the door for her to the lobby and ushered her inside. Twenty more steps and we were in their dining room, which could easily pass for any restaurant in any small town. We sat down at the guest table and imagine who walked in just then – Denise! *"What are YOU doing here?!"* my mother asked, practically squealing like a little girl. And not missing a beat, Denise replied *"This is my favorite place for lunch. Wait until you taste everything!"*

Lunch was served, and as we all three made light conversation, the intake manager stopped by our table to introduce herself. *"Everything was just wonderful,"* my mother offered up brightly. I made their introductions and we chatted about the beautiful day and the flowers in the courtyard. Everyone was lovely. My mother was simply lovely. And she'd made the cut.

The move from Serenity Home was much like the move *to* Serenity Home, only made a little easier since Mom was still mad at their day shift caregiver for some recent scolding. Since things hadn't gotten any better there after the letters, I used it to my advantage. *"You shouldn't have to take that kind of treatment. Let's find a better place to stay while we wait for Dale's vacation time to be approved. Besides, The Community Resting Place is on the map so he can find you! Serenity Home isn't."* This made perfect sense to her.

Robert and I packed her two dressers and moved her bed over to TCRP while Mom was out on her walk with Denise. We only needed to repeat the Dale story a dozen times before she was totally fine with being there. I bought her several new sets of clothes for her to wear for her new friends, hung her paintings all around her room, and put her favorite Walmart quilt – the one she told anyone who commented on it that she'd sewn it herself – on her bed.

I stayed for the evening meal that first night and flipped through magazines with her in the living room afterward. Her new thing was to point at pictures and name each one, like, *"Oh look, a kitchen. And a bird. That's a big dog."* I wonder now if she could sense she was losing her memory and was intentionally reminding herself what things were. Or maybe she was simply happy and relieved to see things she still recognized. Either way, I sat with her and agreed with everything she drew my attention to, like a parent sitting with her child's favorite new picture book.

When I felt like I'd stayed long enough to settle her in, I began constructing excuses to go home. I started with, *"It's getting late Mom, I should probably go so you can get some rest."* Without missing a beat, she looked up, *"I'm not tired,"* and returned to pointing out images on the pages. She added, *"You can sleep here tonight."* When I countered with, *"There's no room for me in your bedroom to stay the night,"* she lobbed right back, *"I'll sleep on the floor."*

My armpits began to sweat as that now familiar sense of panic washed over me. I was everything at once – exhausted from the move, bored with the mindless photo-naming, and impatient to leave. All the while my heart was breaking for my mother who was grasping at ways to keep me there while I busily maneuvered my escape. I was the lowliest human. How could I leave this sad little peanut who was so confused and probably terrified to be left alone in this foreign place? And still I went.

How do I describe the incessant inner conflict I battled when it came to my mother? I won't lie to you and recite that adage, "My mind wanted one thing, but my heart wanted another." Mine both wanted pretty much the same thing – my old mother back and the new one *gone*. Where was the one who loved her youngest daughter and knew without any doubt that I would do anything to keep her safe and cared for? My heart didn't like this new one, and my mind most certainly didn't want this to be happening – to her or to me.

I'd say they both balanced the enormous amount of guilt and obligation I carried pretty equally. I didn't share with anyone the true conflict going on inside me. I still attended my

AA meetings and continued to present stories and seek advice, but I kept this shameful part of me to myself.

I functioned on a level based on my interpretation of what a good daughter should do, but not what a loving one would. My visits were borne from a need to ensure my mother was safe. If I missed a day, the anxiety I suffered was nearly unbearable. But I rarely experienced the feeling of longing for my mother's actual company, and I was very aware of its absence. The emotional punishment I handed down to myself for that was relentless.

I wish I'd had someone to tell me not to worry so much. I felt like an unfeeling machine, but I should have instead focused on the fact that I was stepping up and ensuring my loved one was cared for during a terrible, incredibly uncertain time in her life. But I never shared my good person/bad person quandary with anyone, so how could they?

A friend of mine caught me in line at the post office one day and we ended up out on the sidewalk chatting by our cars. Her mother was in a care facility after having a debilitating stroke and was pleading to go home. We stood on that sidewalk for nearly an hour, both leaning in as we tried to eradicate the other's guilt. She told me her doctor advised her that her only goal while caring for her mother was to manage her quality of *care* – not her quality of *life*. The two might seem the same, but he explained that good care is the only thing we can control at this point in their lives.

I wrote that down on a post-it note when I got home and stuck it to my bathroom mirror. I must've read that quote a dozen times before I finally began to understand it. With my mother, no amount of effort could guarantee a pleasant visit, enjoyable outing, or even appreciated meal. But I could absolutely ensure that she received that visit from me, had that bath, and was properly fed. And that was going to have to be enough for me.

$\mathcal{H}$ER POOR MIS-FIRING BRAIN.

Mom's daily routine at The Community Resting Place established itself quickly, and she seemed to adjust nicely. Up at 7am with a cup of coffee *"just the way she liked it"* brought to her by the morning caregiver. How nice is that? Breakfast at 8:30am with everything she loved – scrambled eggs, toast, maybe a banana, and orange juice – and more coffee, please.

There was an exercise class at 10am three days a week, balanced by Bingo the other two days. Tuesdays were "bus trip days" at 11am. My mother was first on the signup sheet for the eight-seat passenger van driven by a retired volunteer named Fred, and a friend of Robert's. Fay became Fred's favorite because she liked to sit up front and chat. I remember Fred's expression when I connected the dots for him that Fay was my mother, and he then realizing that *I was that daughter.*

It didn't take long for my first "call of concern" to come in from the facility. By Mom's second week there, it was clear that she was quite noncompliant when it came to shower time. Their "Shower Lady" had tried everything to entice Fay into the bathing room, from descriptions of hot sudsy goodness to the promise of her favorites, a banana and hot coffee, afterward.

A common story in my AA meetings often revolved around a loved one's aversion to or even complete disregard for their own personal hygiene. For my mother, that included just about everything except her hair. She couldn't be coerced into the tub or convinced to brush her teeth, but she insisted she needed a perm and a roller-set several times a day, every day.

Her new tube of Colgate remained untouched weeks after arriving at TCRP, and just try locating her toothbrush. I would find it in her walking boots, her flower vase, and even wedged under her TV set. No amount of questioning, suggesting, or offering to help with it could move her to crack that tube open. And her breath stank. I mean, terribly.

I would consciously inhale a breath before getting too close to her, which I didn't do often, since invading Fay's newly developed physical boundaries secured me a 50/50 chance of getting swatted. So most times I just ruffled her hair and dodged her hand shooting up to snatch hold of my wrist.

It was agreed that staff would continue with their well proven tactics and persuade her into the bath. Surely my mother would eventually concede, they reasoned, and everyone could relax. I was only too happy to get off that call, knowing what I did about my mother's obstinate side, and leave everything in their confident, willing hands.

To: Carolyn
From: Ginny

Guess where Fay was when I got to TCRP today?? She was getting A SHOWER! I waited out in the lobby, talking to Emma (always sitting in the same chair). Fay came out with wet crimped hair, looking mad as a hornet and a bit confused. I convinced her to let me set her hair, and by the time I left she had gray Shirley Temple curls all over.

Today we met Lilly & Wanda, both in the new sunroom at the end of the hall. Heard all about how Lilly used to ride a horse to school in Montana when she was young. Wanda it turns out is Fay's bathroom-mate through the adjoining door. Fay has sworn it's a man through that door, which is why she repeatedly locks it from her side and thus locking poor Wanda out of the toilet. Oh, and we met Rubin, who seems nice, but watch out for him. He made it a point of rolling his wheelchair right up to Fay's end of the couch.

Fay always wants to come to the car when Jeff picks me up, because of our Molly-kissing tradition. I always make Jeff wait until I see her re-enter the building before we leave, however. Glad she's getting used to where she lives.

Fay today: "They make me shower here – ONCE A WEEK!" said with indignation.

To: Ginny
From: Carolyn

Her poor mis-firing brain. She's still adjusting to her new surroundings. I love how you handle her. I meant to ask you why you're bringing your own tea bags? I was told it's fine for us to use the coffee and tea they make available in the dining room. Mom hasn't associated the coffee cart with free coffee yet. Just wait! Every time I'm there I offer her some and she's always surprised it's there. I'll pick up an umbrella and some gloves (Damn, I donated so many gloves to the thrift store!) for your poor-weather walks.

I probably forgot to tell you that I reported Mom's overhead sink light malfunction and they fixed it. She showed Denise her magazine stash in her drawers today. I'll have to figure out how to get them back to the living room without becoming the focus of her wrath. I'm surprised she remembered me bringing her all those outfits – aren't they cute?! I labeled them all in front of her, which she seemed to like. Now all she has to do is actually wear them. I'd much prefer she re-discover her toothbrush, but that's another battle. She did tell me that they made an awfully big deal about showers there. And that she didn't see why she had to bathe so often. I told her, "Just like you always said to us kids – a bath once a week whether you need it or not!" (Our Saturday night baths for church on Sunday.)

Thank you for bringing her a puzzle. I left all her puzzles at Serenity Home when I packed her things. I'm glad you found her in the living room! That's so much better than sitting alone in her room. I caught her sitting in her recliner in the dark the other day, sucking grape jelly out of a packet stolen from the dining room. She's now a thief.

While my mother was settling into her own routines at TCRP, the two of us forged ours as well. Mondays became a standing date for us again, this time with Bowling Day. Not the traditional trip to the bowling alley – more the unroll the oil cloth lane, set the plastic pins at the end, then throw the rubber bowling ball as hard as you can at the poor pin-setting kid at the end, times ten.

One of our town's private life skills schools brought a group of students each week as part of their volunteer curriculum requirement to set up, keep score, and break down the bowling set. I made a big deal of getting the residents excited when I saw the van pull into the parking lot. Those kids would burst through the front doors at precisely 3pm and be greeted with a hearty round of cheers. It was fun to get the group revved and equally rewarding to see the grins on the students' faces as they received their enthusiastic reception.

They were in this particular school because of severe socialization deficiencies and behavioral issues, so it was particularly heartwarming to see them carefully interact and maneuver among the elderly residents. Their shy sideways glances eventually transformed into full-on grins and careful pats on the backs of those eccentric old folks whose main goal it seemed was to ride those kids and prod a response out of them.

Predictably, the girls resembled any number of daughters, granddaughters, or even themselves – *"I used to look just like her,"* and the boys invariably became the objects of outlandish flirting. Emma loved every boy that came through the front doors, often pinching them on their backsides if they passed within reach of her wheelchair. And Mom had something to say about every girl's outfit. *"Just look at her! Who would let their daughter leave the house looking like that?"* she'd bellow with no care as to who heard her.

More than once, I'd lock eyes with some unfortunate girl

and make a face to show her I knew my mother was crazy. *"If you don't have something nice to say..."* had flown out the window, and now no one was exempt. The fact that I was being pardoned for a short while as she focused her disapproval on someone new did little to console me.

Maybe I could've laughed off our new and disparate mother/daughter role if only I'd found that one perfect book, gone to that extra meeting, or had one more meaningful conversation with just the right person, but I don't know. All I could do was compare this Fay with the mother who raised me to hold my tongue when it was about to issue something critical, and I couldn't make sense of it. It was ugly. She was ugly. And I struggled simply to stay at her side those days.

But those Mondays saved me, much like Lunch Days had. They provided a reliable hour for us to focus on something outside ourselves and keep the conversation from sinking into *"Why am I here and when is Dale coming to get me?"* quicksand.

As rousing as those afternoons began, though, the atmosphere in the room always seemed to dwindle midway through the game, and I could sense the attention of the bowlers drifting. We were constantly herding residents to line up for the next frame. Some would absent-mindedly wander off, and others fell asleep in their chairs.

I decided to shake things up a little by offering prizes for first, second, and third place winners on our next bowling day. Just a little something to make the high scorers feel rewarded and special, and maybe coax some of the nonparticipants to join in. On my way to bowling the following Monday, I ran to the thrift store and snagged a teddy bear, teacup, and porcelain photo frame. I couldn't contain my excitement as I placed all three prizes on the table and announced to the group that today was "Bowling with Prizes" day.

"So bowl your best! Hey William, I heard you used to bowl.

Want to join the group and maybe win a prize?"

Everyone skuttled over to the table to see what they might win, fingering the teacup and squeezing the bear. Between turns I'd congratulate a handsome strike or neat spare and remind them they might be in line for a fabulous prize, to which I'd hear, *"What prize? I didn't see any prizes."*

At the end of the final frame, our student scorekeeper tallied up the points and announced that Fay (what are the chances?) came in first place. Applause!! As I ushered her to the prize table to choose from the three on display, I heard, *"Hey! She gets the best prize because her daughter is here!"* Lilly came in second, but she wanted Fay's prize and so refused to choose either of the two remaining. Grace, who came in third, walked straight over to my mother and snatched the teacup (Fay's chosen prize) out of her lap. Two caregivers were out of their seats in seconds, separating and distracting the three very angry ladies as I quietly removed all three prizes and stuffed them into my purse before anyone noticed.

"Bowling with Prizes" promptly became "Bowling with Cookies," and the following Monday *everyone* received a healthy cookie, pre-approved by the dietician.

It didn't take long for the first complaint, *"Boy, you'd think we'd get some coffee to go with these dry cookies."* And just like that, "Bowling with Cookies" turned into "Bowling with Cookies and Coffee," presenting me with an entirely new set of challenges. It seemed each resident had their own favorite (if not peculiar) way of enjoying their coffee. There was black, of course, *"Just like I like my..."* "William!" Various shades of cream and packets of sweetener, *"No, Phyllis, I can't give you four sugars with your diabetes, you know that."* And the prize for most unusual (don't say "prize!"), *"Half coffee and half tea, please, and don't forget the ice cube."*

With a cookie deposited in everyone's lap, I'd sprint toward the coffee station repeating the list of requests that were fresh in my head. As I dispensed each personalized cup, a new problem sprang up. Seemed I had three cunning residents among the group who could manage to eat an entire cookie while I filled coffee orders, consume a second cookie as I passed out cups, because *"You forgot to give me a cookie,"* and once everyone had their cup, complain they never got a cookie in the first place to enjoy with their coffee. Call it cunning or call it forgetful, it only took me two Mondays to change my tactics and take the coffee orders *before* doling out the cookies.

There were Mondays when the kids didn't come, and those were the days I panicked. They might have been on vacation, or their class schedule didn't allow for a bowling trip, but none of that mattered to the disappointed residents.

The mood in the main room dipped noticeably low, and I suddenly felt the responsibility to fill that time with the entire expectant group, not just my mother. I'd do about anything to avoid an uncomfortable, awkward visit that involved fielding a plethora of questions about why she was there, what had happened to her house, and when was Dale coming. I had well practiced answers for everything, but the tone of our visit went deep south on those days, and it left me drained, unsettled, and depressed.

One of my solutions to those empty Mondays was Carolyn's Nail Salon. *"Take a seat ladies! Have a cookie and tell me your story while I make your nails beautiful,"* I'd singsong as women giggling like little girls jockeyed for position in line. It was an easy way to kill an hour or so while making everyone feel pretty. And the stories they told! Lilly's back was killing her because she'd just ridden her horse that morning and they'd jumped a fence. Wanda still wasn't speaking to her daughter because she was dating an Indian (What in the world do I say to that?!). And Janice had decided to leave her husband and run away with her lover, whom she waited for every day in the front room.

The first nails to be done were always my mother's, and she would remain seated next to me the rest of the time, blowing on them as instructed. It was acknowledged by all that she was first because she was the "honorary mother," and she

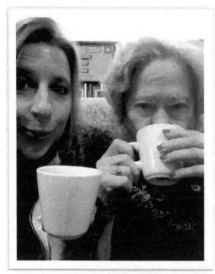

~ *Fay, her Slut Red nails and eighth cup of decaf* ~

loved that I made a big deal about it as the rest busily arranged the order of their chairs. They'd maneuver in one by one for a light file, a coat of clear, and a color.

Picking colors became a game because they could never decide on one, and I needed to speed things along or they'd have wet nails at the dinner table. So I started giving them names like Passion Pink, Virgin Blush, and Slut Red. My mother would act like she was going to faint each time I named them off, but the ladies loved it and laughed like crazy, asking me to repeat the list again, even though I'd just done it for the client before them. Each time, Mom would position her wrist up against her temple, throw her head back in a perfect swoon, and they'd crack up all over again.

On the Mondays when the residents met me in the front room with, *"We're not bowling today! They're not coming! But we just did our nails! There's nothing to do!"* we had "Carolyn's Concert Day." Keeping them happy and occupied had become more than just a challenge to me. My own visits with my mother could be measured by the overall mood of the group, so I stayed motivated. I began keeping my ukulele in the back seat of my truck for just these days. I'm a self-taught, below average player, and my singing is consistently flat, but it was a great hour of practice, and they really loved music.

I even learned some church hymns to play for them after discovering that the alternating church choirs usually played to a full house every Sunday. An advantage to playing for this group was that I could start right over with the same songs when I got to the end of my list. No one even noticed. We'd belt out Johnny Cash's "Do Lord" and "This Little Light of Mine," sometimes three and four times. They even knew the words to Norman Greenbaum's "Spirit in the Sky," singing out when we got to, *"I got a friend in Jesus."*

One day I was strumming away and feeling proud that I'd gotten through a tricky set of chords when I heard Lilly on the couch shout-whisper to Janice, *"That girl couldn't carry a tune if she had one in her back pocket,"* to which Janice bobbed her head in agreement and the two tittered together as they clapped along to the beat. Thank goodness I'd already spent several years in Fay Land by then, with plenty of AA meetings, resource books, and Prozac under my belt to glide right over any hurt feelings. I told myself Lilly was no different than my mother with her missing filter, and besides, who could dispute it?

Life seemed to be evening out for my mother and me. For my mother, because she had so much more structure in her daily routine and people to interact with, which generally kept her too busy to get into trouble, and for me, the exact same reasons. But as cliches go, "Nothing lasts forever," and more accurately, "The honeymoon is over."

CONFLICT BETWEEN HEAD AND HEART.

Year Four – Stage 4
(Mild Dementia)

Fay was granted a fair amount of leeway as she navigated her "getting used to" period at TCRP. The staff were prepared to work around the disorientation and even panic a new resident typically experienced upon arrival, and my mother was no exception. The intake coordinator was pleased with how quickly she acclimated to most of the new routines and personalities that suddenly surrounded her. Showers remained a special challenge, but I only heard about them in passing during my visits anymore, *"Boy, your mother must be made of sugar!"* and then turning to Fay, *"You're worried you're going to melt, aren't you sweetie!"*

And much like bell curves do, her behaviors that seemed manageable along the plateaued top side of the bell lasted for many months. Long enough, really, to trick me into thinking this was as bad as it was going to get. But somewhere along the line she became progressively more challenging as she rounded out the back side and began her rapid descent. Like a simmering pot of pasta right before you place the lid on and walk away "for only a minute," her downward slide at TCRP mimicked the first sputters under the tinkling lid and escalated to the point of erupting over the sides and scorching the burners. And that's when the calls started.

"Hello, Carolyn? This is the administrator at TCRP. Your

mother has been taking food off her table mates' plates and eating it, so we had to move her to an isolated table."

- An isolated table? By herself? She'll feel terrible! (And Isolated!) Is there another table you could move her to with more active residents? Ones who'd be unlikely to let her near their plates?

So Fay was moved to a livelier table where any attempts to snatch a sandwich would've been met with the stab of a fork. She promptly stopped stealing food from her neighbors and she enjoyed it much better anyway.

"Hi Carolyn, it's the administrator at TCRP. Sorry for another call so soon. Your mom was found in the kitchen by herself today. She'd emptied the refrigerator and both freezers and arranged everything onto the counters. We're just lucky we caught her in time."

- Is there any way to keep the kitchen door locked when staff isn't in the kitchen?

And Fay became officially locked out of the kitchen whenever staff left for the day. These calls continued, sometimes in rapid succession and sometimes with weeks separating them.

I think my first truly alarming call came in the form of, *"Your mother let herself out the hallway exit door in the middle of the night last night and a police officer brought her back... in her nightgown."*

All exit doors were kept unlocked for emergency exit safety, and although they chimed when opened, staff didn't hear them open around 1am when Mom made her escape. She wandered across the street and over to the hospital, entering through their double doors. The night nurse asked if she could help her, to which Fay replied she didn't know where she was.

It didn't take much to connect the dots when a lost, elderly woman presented herself in her nightgown after midnight that she probably belonged across the street, and so the receptionist called the police for an escort. How much do I love my little town? Let me count the ways. And it was an easy fix for TCRP: they attached a few noise makers on the door handle in case she tried it again. Their theory was the rattling noise makers would either jar her into a more conscious state or at least do a better job of alerting nighttime staff.

"Truly Alarming Call Number Two" came a few weeks later when I was informed that Mom had gone rogue for the afternoon. She'd apparently scaled the courtyard fence unnoticed and taken herself for a walk. A neighbor on the other end of the block recognized her, and not seeing Denise or Ginny, went out to inquire where her walking partners were. He discovered that Mom was alone and quite pleased with herself, but very lost and thirsty. The nice neighbor gave her an orange Gatorade, which pleased her *very* much, and asked if he could join her on her walk. He steered her back toward TCRP and suggested they go inside to see what it was like inside, clever man.

Easy fix Part Two: a brand new, taller fence was installed (they reassured me that a new one had been planned for a while and was currently in the budget). The new fence came with a mounted gate pad and a tricky four-digit code – 1234 – just the right amount of difficulty to thwart my wily mother.

I was beginning to have a Pavlov's-dog-like response to calls from The Community Resting Place – only instead of hungry saliva at the signal of food, mine was a constrictive tightening in the chest followed by a swift blast of panic sweat. It was just another example of the conflict between my head and my heart when it came to my mother – *Oh shit, it's TCRP – don't answer the phone. Oh shit, it's TCRP – trip over yourself as you lunge for the phone.* I became quickly conditioned to dread their calls and to brace myself for the next new calamity. As much as I didn't want to answer each call, I equally couldn't resist my need to know immediately what was happening with my mother.

There were more calls and more small catastrophes over the next few years, each one advancing in severity and urgency. In the earlier Fay Days, she was caught hoarding meat from the dinner table in her drawers. It didn't take them long to find the source of decaying stench in her room, but it did result in another call.

> **To:** Carolyn
> **From:** Ginny
>
> I'll see your jelly-sucking story and raise you one. I went to Volunteer Day at TCRP today – I saw Denise there, too. When I first came in, I spotted Fay scurrying to her room, full of purpose, holding a precious bundle wrapped in napkins. When I intercepted her and said hi she had this look like she'd been busted. Then I figured it out – she was squirreling away food to her room. Someday a thorough drawer search might be in order (of course when she's not present!) as I do believe you may find spoiling food. She had cookies this time. Ten minutes later she was again headed to her room, hunched over another bundle. I asked Denise how many trips she'd made so far that day, and she'd only counted three...

She'd also begun filling her dressers with every magazine she could find in the living area, writing "Fay" in huge letters on each cover, until she couldn't fit her underwear in her drawers anymore and the magazine racks were empty out front. Each time a staff member attempted to retrieve the magazines she would launch into a tirade over them coming into her room and stealing from her, just like her daughter. In fact, it was her daughter who had been stealing the magazines from the living room, so she had to hide them in her drawers to protect them. Thus resulting in yet another call from TCRP.

> **To:** Carolyn
> **From:** Ginny
>
> Once again Fay pulled her extensive magazine collection out of her many drawers to show me what you'd done.

She offered some to me initially, but after I said I'd take a few (to secretly return to the living room), I must have become suspicious to her, and so she waited until I wasn't looking to stuff them all back in her drawers. Oh, and you are no longer Queen Latifa the cover model, but in the past week you have been (I am not kidding): Eva Longoria, Courtney Cox, Jillian Michaels, and Princess Kate The Duchess of Cornwall. She tells everyone, so be ready for autographs.

Another new development I've watched is that she has been taking on the role of caretaker for the others in the TCRP (have I mentioned this to you yet?). Yesterday she approached Glynda, slouched and sleepy on the couch, took her hand in a very caring manner and introduced herself. Glynda was confused and asked who Fay was, and Fay told her that she takes care of her (which I believe *unfortunately and to the dismay of real staff*, is true). Fay went on to show Glynda where she (Fay) sits on the other couch and told Glynda she has been working at TCRP for two years. I can imagine the wheels turning fast in Fay's head as she makes up some of her stories.

I wish I could say that seeing "The Community Resting Place" light up on my phone screen affected me less with each call, but it never did. In fact, I assigned them a special ring tone so I would recognize them immediately and instantly take the call. I'd even developed the habit of going to bed with my phone charging on my nightstand so I wouldn't miss a midnight call. It didn't matter that the news was almost always bad, I simply couldn't bear the thought of not knowing what was happening to my mother.

I remember receiving a particularly panicked call one day from the shift supervisor, who explained that Fay had lost her bridge, and she was introducing herself to everyone with a large, toothless grin. It was upsetting other residents, and they asked me to come help search her room for it, since she was refusing entrance to anyone else but me (a huge surprise, since I was usually barred).

I arrived to find her in the living room, moving from one

person to the next, leaning in and baring her creepy, gaping smile. She seemed to be enjoying everyone's discomfort, or maybe this new gummy sensation in her mouth was something so incredible that she wanted to share it, who knows. When asked where her six-tooth apparatus was, she simply couldn't begin to know.

She followed us to her room, and I began methodically removing all the rotting fruit and magazines from her drawers while two caregivers sat with her on the bed, hands fidgeting and humming her nervous non-tune. She didn't like that they'd summoned me (she'd already forgotten that she'd requested my presence), and she especially didn't like me rooting through her things.

"Leave those alone! They're mine! You've already taken everything else I own, now you want these?"

I watched her expression flip-flop between confusion and rage as I searched her coats, shoes, and finally moved on to her pants, all the while calmly reassuring her that we only wanted to help her find her teeth. My poor little bird only knew that she was being violated by her daughter and that her possessions were likely about to be confiscated from her as well. Meanwhile, I was just as furious with her for losing her bridge as I struggled with the heartbreak of witnessing my mother's sincere feelings of helplessness.

I checked every pocket and found only folded Kleenex, crumpled Kleenex, and spoiled food bound by Kleenex. I'd run out of hiding places and was ready to end my search when I remembered Roxanne's lost FedEx package with Mom's ID in it. And I found it. She'd jammed it between her mattresses along the back wall, wrapped inside a sock.

Her shock was genuine as it tumbled out of the sock and into my palm, all the while demanding we find who had done this dirty deed.

We were lucky. The dentist saw her the next day and was able to successfully reinstall it, although he warned me it was going to be a short-lived fix, given the poor condition of Fay's anchor teeth. I decided this temporary solution was the best route for now, avoiding a full-on denture installment involving tooth removal and another apparatus that could easily be lost. In the meantime, we'd all happily returned a much more acceptable smile on my mother's face.

Fay didn't always lose things, though; sometimes she found things. I remember coming through the lobby doors one day and greeting the regulars who sat along the front wall in their self-assigned seats. My mother had just exited her room and was walking down the hall toward me sporting a pair of bright yellow, wire rimmed glasses. She looked like John Lennon, and I had to laugh as I complimented her on them, *"What? You act like you've never seen me in glasses."* No one knew where they'd come from or what had happened to her real glasses, but she wasn't in distress or bumping into walls, so we continued as though nothing unusual had happened. Eventually, the yellow glasses also disappeared, and Fay carried on without any at all.

To: Carolyn
From: Ginny

When I arrived today to get Fay for our walk, she was in her room with the lights out. I turned on the lamp and she hissed (YES, HISSED!) at me, so I opened her blinds and cracked the window while I was at it (smells like rotted cheese in there). I commented that her new haircut looked good, and she replied she hadn't gotten a haircut, then looked in the mirror to see if what I'd said was true. We chatted a bit, then left for a walk. First we checked out the gardens in back. Fay proclaimed she had never seen them before (we start every walk there). Jay was out there in his one-piece jumpsuit, tending to things, and I introduced Fay like I do every time. He reminds her that his is the room right next to hers every time, but he doesn't make a big deal of it.

Today I had to repeat the storyline that this move was so Dale could find her better, and that it was a big bonus that it seems to be such an upgrade.

I continued to second-guess every decision I made those days. My attempt at a solution oftentimes only made the situation worse. And equally often, my decision to let something ride and sort itself out ended as badly as if I'd tried to fix it. What happened to me?! I was the girl who could confidently make buying and selling recommendations for my real estate clients. I could walk through a worn out building and see exactly how to renovate it back to its former glory. But when it came to caring for my mother my confidence level sat at zero. Instead, I forged ahead with each new disaster, desperately grasping at some semblance of control over what felt like a constantly moving target.

And she was changing. Her obsession with money disappeared practically overnight. I don't know where all the dollar bills and change she kept in her pocket ever ended up, but one day it was all gone, and she never mentioned it again. Same with the telephone in her room. She never did dial anyone, and calls seemed to aggravate her more and more, with *"Some man keeps calling me and checking up on me, and he knows where I live!"* So I happily removed the $34 basic service plan from the list of Fay-bills I'd been juggling.

Even painting her fingernails was different from before. I remember one day after a couple of years of doing them, I had just painted her last one and she was dutifully blowing on them when a staff member wandered by and commented on her pretty red nails. Dead serious, she replied, *"Thank you, I had them done last week."*

To: Carolyn
From: Denise

Fay's doing well these days. No "I want to go home" at all today. Forgot to mention that Fay's new thing is she tells me she hears your voice all around TCRP but in her next breath, do you ever drop in to visit her? Why no! :O

Denise and I discovered around the same time that Fay had become the resident man-eater at TCRP. Whether it was the maintenance man or someone else's husband, she simply loved men and gravitated toward them. To be fair, every new male resident was fair game for about half a dozen of the more mobile ladies, but *my* mother always seemed to sit the closest and smile the brightest, inevitably landing herself a steady supply of boyfriends. Each new tryst was relatively short lived, however, since the male residents sadly seemed to cycle out much faster than the female residents.

To: Carolyn
From: Ginny

Fay and I came in from our walk today, and as we were walking down the long hallway, we saw Roy in his favorite red plaid shirt way up ahead. We eventually caught up to him, and as Fay approached him from behind, she took her mittens off and very deliberately pinched one of his ass cheeks through his pants. A real pinch, low and centered, nothing mild about it. I was caught off guard – too late to stop it. Roy's deep furrowed brow as he turned around said it all – he was *pisssssed,* before AND after he saw Fay's elfish ear-to-ear grin. A staff member saw and handled it very well by explaining to Fay that she needed to make sure to never do that again, that it wasn't appropriate. Fay seemed to take it in stride. I felt a little guilty, maybe like I should have stopped her, but it happened too fast and had me so stunned.

Another problem you may have noticed is with Fay's room temperature – she is constantly messing with the buttons, the temp gets cold, she blames someone for coming into her room. The temp gets hot, she blames someone for coming into her room. I'm always changing those buttons to keep it ok in there.

To: Carolyn
From: Ginny

Fay was in Roy's room again, watching TV, so I guess her butt-pinching infraction was forgiven. Later, Roy came out to sing hymns with the visiting church choir.

When Fay spotted him she pointed him out to me, calling him "Archie." (Former husband/boyfriend?) He joined us on the couch, Fay nestled in close to him to share the hymnbook. She called him Archie one more time, but he didn't correct her.

Fay is back to helping Glynda up out of the couch to her walker again. Before I could try to dissuade her, a staff member stopped her, explaining to Fay that she might hurt herself. Fay bristled and gave a snappy retort (as I've witnessed on more than one occasion when staff need to firm up boundaries).

Roy was Mom's first love-loss, and it unsettled everyone, presenting a particular dilemma for staff with, *"What will we tell Fay?"* How were they going to tell her that she'd lost her Dr. Oz-watching buddy? Or that she was going to be sitting alone on the couch this Sunday during church services? There was some discussion, and they finally decided not to say anything and instead kept a close eye on her that day. It only took one or two trips down the hall to Roy's newly emptied room before she returned to the main living room and picked up as usual with no other mention of him – or of Ben after that, or Marvin still later.

It was as if these lovely gentlemen came into her life but completely disappeared from her memory once they were gone. My mother's lack of short-term memory proved to be a Godsend for her, if not a little unnerving for us. While we were relieved she didn't suffer the pain of loss with each departure, it left us monumentally aware of her emotional imbalance as we suffered the loss for her instead.

Hiding the Fact that She Wasn't Recognizing Me

Year Five – Stage 5, a little 6
(Moderate/Moderately Severe Dementia)

My mother's dementia continued to advance. I rarely detected a noticeable change during my regular visits, but a vacation or my return from our winter spent in Florida would leave me stunned by her progression. I'd enter the room after having been gone several weeks or months and scan the couches for her. My eyes would land on her, and I'd inhale a calming breath before I approached her, taking in all the changes.

Her entire head seemed to be shrinking. I was sure I could cup her tiny skull into my palm like the apple head dolls we used to make as kids. Her face was creased in every direction with lines so deep they looked like someone had drawn them on with a brown crayon. Those were the visits when the changes were so startling to me that I had to turn my head and carefully wipe at my tears so she wouldn't see. Mother Nature was still manipulating me, but this time instead of rewarding me for returning, she seemed to be preparing me for my mother's departure.

She'd begun pausing when she stood up to adjust her shirt over her pants. It took several times before I realized she wasn't actually adjusting anything, just settling her balance, which I suppose she thought she was concealing from anyone who might be watching. I'm still amazed that my mother could have the presence of mind to disguise her need to steady herself with this wardrobe adjustment when she couldn't even remember what she had for lunch, or that she'd even *had* lunch.

She was also nodding off in her chair during my visits now – oftentimes mid-sentence. I'd be telling her a story and out she'd go, chin to chest, arms folded across her belly. Eventually her head would bob back up and she'd focus her eyes on the room, look at me, and behave as if nothing had happened. And of course, so would I.

> **To:** Carolyn
> **From:** Ginny
>
> I was in Fay's room today, door closed, talking to her when "RapRapRap!" on the door – it was her suitor/ friend Marvin all dressed nice for a drop-in visit. He seemed surprised that I was there, and we invited him in, but this was near the end of my visit, so I didn't talk to him long. Funny, his name came up during my walk with Fay outside earlier today. The conversation went something like this:
>
> Fay: "I don't have a husband anymore"
> Me: "I know Fay, I'm sorry. Sal sounds like he was a great husband."
> Fay: "I wouldn't even know how to be married again"
> Me: <admittedly digging a little> "Marvin seems like a nice guy, <joking> you never know if he'll catch you off guard & pop the question..."
> Fay (with indignation): "Well if he did <stuttering> I'd...I'd tell him I have to think it over!"

There were some days my mother would greet me with a polite, *"Hello,"* as I approached her, and it wouldn't be until I bent to ruffle her hair and say, *"Hello MeeMaw! I've come to see you!"* that she would do a double-take and exclaim, *"Oh! What did you do with your hair! (makeup!) (clothes!) You look so different!"* It was another excuse she'd devised to hide the fact that she wasn't recognizing me every time I came for a visit, just like she did with her balance adjustments. Were there studies on how a person with dementia compensates for the forgetfulness they experience? How can they compensate when they don't know what it is they're forgetting in the first place?

I'd read an article about it online on a site called, "A Place for Mom." It identified five ways the elderly hide signs of dementia, like refusing to participate in activities they once loved because they can't remember how to do them, covering up mishaps like overdrawn accounts or poor driving, normalizing unusual behaviors with, "I'm fine, I'm just tired," being "too busy" to care about their appearance, and forgetting holidays and important dates because, "they lost their calendar." I was amazed to find my mother in each of the five ways listed.

Some days I'd arrive confident and upbeat, and I'd play around with her to see if I could identify any movement in her stages (and it broke the monotony of pointing at pictures in magazines). I could gauge her willingness to answer questions by her mood when I sat down. I might start by asking her what she had for breakfast. If she quipped right back that she hadn't eaten because they're punishing her, I'd know my game was going to be short lived. If I asked her if she lived there, she'd say, *Of course not! I live in New York!*" Where her past 20 years in Georgia had gone, I couldn't tell you.

As long as I posed my questions conversationally, she'd play along. But if I asked whether she remembered my name or what year it was, she'd immediately go silent, jaw jutted forward, and the game would be over. She could still tell the difference between a casual chat and a test.

It was her newest habit of standing up mid-conversation and disappearing down the hall to her room that marked a turning point for me. The first time it happened, I figured she needed to use the bathroom and was being modest about announcing it. When 20 minutes went by, I crept to her room to see what was taking her so long and peeked in. She was sitting on her bed and humming her non-tune, immersed in her magazines and surrounded by gaping dresser drawers. Eyes wide, a thunderbolt of realization struck me that she'd completely forgotten our visit (mid-visit!).

If freedom had a scent, I could smell it just then. *"This is really happening! No more anxiously fabricated excuses to leave! Run!"* reverberated through my head. I sucked in my breath and jerked backwards out of the doorway, praying she wouldn't look up from her stash. I'd just been given a glimpse into my immediate future and the new-found liberation I'd been handed made me almost giddy. I breezed out the double doors after waving goodbye to all the ladies perched along the front wall, telling THEM I'd see them tomorrow.

To: Carolyn
From: Ginny

Fay was again quite disoriented after we went on our walk today. I'm starting to wonder how others (Denise, staff) handle it. It's as if the slate is wiped clean each time she leaves the building and returns, and she has to be reminded that TCRP is where she lives. Today I needed to be much more direct. She was so insistent that she didn't live there, and she was getting pissed that she couldn't leave with me (like I was abandoning her). She put her hat back on & everything. I had to think fast and tell her that Jeff and I were going to a friend's house for dinner. I told her that she has a room here and this is where she stays until other arrangements can be made, but she seemed unconvinced. I'm a little wary of walking with her now if it's upsetting her :/. Ideas?

To: Ginny
From: Carolyn

Mom's dementia is progressing, for sure. Today she told me, "Marvin lives down the block, but how can I go visit him if you don't show me how to get there?" So I showed her how to get down the hall. She took off in that direction and I let her go. I waited ten minutes and left – it's her new thing. She just leaves me and forgets about me. She also insists she lives upstairs (on the roof I guess??). She repeatedly asks where I live, if I have a husband, and that neither you nor Denise ever come to walk with her anymore. But then in her next breath she tells me she walks every day. I don't try to help her make that connection because it only makes her mad. Tonight she insisted she did NOT have a tooth pulled today (as she opened her mouth to prove it, revealing a fresh hole and then, surprised, felt around it with her finger.) But then she shut it and didn't say another word about it. Proud to say, neither did I.

Denise's approach seems to suit Mom perfectly. She mock-punches her in the arm and promises she'll be back tomorrow to walk again. Even you can say that, whether you're coming tomorrow or not – because she won't remember either way. I tell her the same thing now because it reassures her. I guess my advice is (and can you believe this is about to come from me???) to take her a whole lot less seriously, tease her, reassure her, suggest she go check in on Marvin...any of that will work. You're my angel.

Things seemed to be moving faster. Her changes were more perceptible. It became increasingly easier for me to leave her after each visit. Her sense of time was distorted now, and I found that I could simply reach over for a quick squeeze or a kiss on the head and chirp, *"OK, Mom! I'm gonna go now and I'll be back tomorrow!"* (Whether I was or wasn't.) My promise to return was really the only thing she needed, so I always gave it. If I visited five days in a row she'd insist that I hadn't been to see her in months. When I returned from a month in Florida she'd smile at me vaguely, I'd remind her who I was, and we'd begin as though I were there yesterday.

Gone were the days when I'd begin preparing my exit strategy well in advance of my departure, inwardly agonizing over what sort of interrogation I'd receive this time. I no longer had to sweat through some story about somewhere I needed to be or the project that had to get done, counting on my mother's working-class mindset to empathize.

To: Carolyn
From: Ginny

Found your mom in her room today. I made a comment about all the magazines she had in her dresser, and she said that you come and leave them all there for her. This being said about one minute after swearing you never come :)

A worker had a bald-headed baby there – her granddaughter, maybe 8 months old. Fay was beside herself as usual, squishing her fat cheeks and kissing her. At one point Fay went to take the baby from the worker's arms and surprisingly (to me at least) they let her! They stood very close, and it was brief, but Fay was overjoyed.

EVERYONE IS FAMILY HERE.

Years Four, Five, and Six

We'd already celebrated a few Thanksgivings and Christ-mases at The Community Resting Place, each holiday with an obscenely large turkey and a million gooey side dishes from contributing family members visiting their respective elders.

They'd become our new tradition, always starting at the same designated time and beginning with the ritual greeting of a sizable portion of our town. These folks whom we knew from interactions we had throughout our days outside of TCRP were now our holiday family. We hugged the check-out lady from Safeway, shook hands with our bank teller, and chatted with the UPS man, unaware until then that they were the daughters/sons/ spouses of one of the little ladies or gents I served cookies and coffee to every Monday after bowling. Unlikely friendships were forged by our newfound connections, and whether we saw each other at The Community Resting Place or out to dinner, there was a gentle understanding between us now that bound us together.

I'll always remember the one Thanksgiving my mother entertained us with a comedy routine she unintentionally choreographed with her fruit punch. I had just brought her a glass and set it beyond her napkin, spill patrol style. She reached for her glass and took a sip as she surveyed her plate of food. Red-faced and choking, she slammed the glass down and grabbed her napkin, sputtering, *"They poisoned the punch! Don't drink it!"* I leaned in and shushed her while sampling the offending punch – tart, but totally benign.

I scooted my chair back and half-rose to go see what else I could get for her, but she reached for my arm and made me sit back down. Even with the gaping holes in Mom's filter (and a possible murder attempt on us all), she still held tight to her daughter's careful upbringing – we didn't make "scenes."

A few bites into her meal, she reached for her glass again and took another sip, only to have that same horrified look return to her face. She leaned into me and handed over her glass, *"Does that taste funny to you?"* she rasped, as I dutifully sampled the poison she'd apparently decided was okay for me to drink. Keeping my expression neutral, I swallowed and shook my head no. She then returned her attention to her plate as if nothing had just happened. After her third visit to her glass, I realized she was operating on a 30 second loop, so I nudged Robert and mouthed, *"Watch."* Within seconds she went back for her punch, took a sip, and immediately followed it with an expression of utter shock and disgust over just how *"devious and wicked the staff were."*

Robert stealthily traded out her punch with a glass of water while I distracted her, and she cleaned her plate with no further mention of espionage. We made it through the rest of the meal without anyone at our table ever becoming privy to Fay's libelous accusations.

Christmas came the following month, of course, and at the exact same time with the same group of people, we enjoyed another massive dinner. But this time, with gifts. It was incredibly heartwarming to see the personalized presents the staff had carefully chosen for every resident, each one based on a specific need or interest. There were puzzles, cologne, pajamas, and sweaters scattered throughout the main room. But the wrapping paper? Most of it could be found neatly folded in each resident's lap, like treasure.

My mother opened a prettily wrapped box containing a

lovely cardigan nestled in gold tissue – with no buttons. The perceptive caregivers were quite aware that Fay had recently become fixated on the buttons of her clothes. No button was safe, and where they disappeared to, no one knew, but every item of clothing she owned was now quite buttonless.

Robert was always a good sport about spending our holidays with my mother and everyone else's family, and I cannot voice loudly enough how loved and supported that made me feel. We still disagreed on so many aspects of managing Fay's care and navigating through all her escapades, but he always embraced her holiday events.

One Christmas, we thought it would be fun for Santa (Robert) and his festively costumed elf (me) to visit after dinner and hand out the gifts that staff usually did. TCRP's administrator agreed that it might be a good idea to keep the residents, sleepy after their large meal, a little more engaged and excited to receive their gifts. We paraded through the family-filled living and dining rooms with Robert booming, *"HO! HO! HO!"* while planting kisses, giving hugs, and shaking hands. Everyone loved Santa, men and women alike, but the resident males *especially* loved Santa's elf. It was a treacherous path I traveled behind Santa passing out candy canes as a random hand would brush my butt. More than once someone made a daring attempt to see what was under my elf-skirt. I think the costume encouraged their bad behavior, because *certainly* I never received that sort of welcome on bowling days when I was Fay's sweet daughter who brought them cookies.

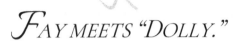

FAY MEETS "DOLLY."

Year Six – Stage 6
(Moderately Severe Dementia)

That same Christmas brought Dolly into my mother's life. I'd been racking my brain for a suitable and memorable (hah!) gift for her. I Googled "appropriate gifts for Alzheimer's patients" and stumbled upon an anatomically correct, appropriately weighted doll with "RealTouch" vinyl skin and hand-rooted hair. "Little Lauren" could be mine for $139 plus shipping and handling. I wasn't thrilled with the price, knowing my chances of her liking it were 50/50, but bells went off as I read the description of how realistic this doll was. And considering the days of anyone handing over their baby to my mother were quickly dwindling, I hoped this little substitution would somehow satisfy her undying mothering instinct.

Should I tell you that she loved that little baby doll? Or that she wouldn't put her down, ever? And should I tell you how happy and relieved I was that I'd finally found something to completely occupy Fay's busy hands for the next several months? Yes, yes I should.

She immediately named her Dolly. It was as if that doll flicked the happiness switch on in my mother's life. She seemed to have a new outlook on everything, as if this little baby needed her and she wasn't going to let her down (or put her down). Ever. She also became alarmingly possessive. As loving as my mother was toward that innocent baby doll, she was a viper toward anyone who came near it. There were regular tiffs and scuffles over the next few weeks that ended in hurt feelings among the other ladies who only wanted to admire and maybe hold Dolly for just a minute or two, and Fay was having none of it.

My mother could now almost always be found seated in a living room chair with Dolly sheltered securely in her lap, donning some newly crocheted dress from who-knows-who. It was touching to see the care being given to her new charge. She treated that doll as if it were her true infant, complete with

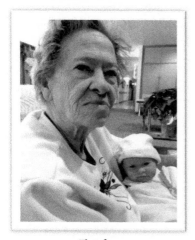

~ That face ~

cooing, rocking, and burping throughout the day. Then one afternoon I arrived to find Dolly sporting a fresh, black tattoo – "FAY" had been written in large capital letters with a Sharpie pen across her entire left foot. Poor defaced Dolly, but I decided it could have been much worse and didn't even ask about it.

Spring came again, signaling the beginning of a new walking season. Denise resumed her morning routine of dropping in from the gym to head out again with Fay, who was always ready for her at the front door – some days with as many as three pairs of pants on and a different shoe on her left foot than on her right. This year there was a noticeable change in Mom's speed and endurance, but not in her determination. Denise reported back to me that she was taking it a lot slower with her and they weren't walking around the full block anymore. I think it was a little sad for both of us. Sad for Denise to witness the change in her walking buddy, and sad for me to know that this was *just another indicator of Mom's certain decline.*

To: Carolyn
From: Denise

Our walk was nice today; the weather was great for it. I try to stay near her because now and then she'll lose her balance/footing a little – this has been happening for a little while. She hasn't fallen or anything, but she's not quite as steady as before... Also, she's consistently confused when we return from our walks, questioning why we're entering the building and asking where her home is. I usually gloss over it and mention whatever it is we're going to do next (like sing hymns with the church choir today), then I ask her permission to put my coat away which is my effort to "ground" her by showing her to her room. We went straight to her room today, and she said several times while pacing, "THIS is my home... THIS is my home." I didn't even bring up the Dale story as I wasn't sure what she was thinking. I just reassured her by saying, "and this is your quilt, and your clothes, and..."

ℋOLDING ONTO MEMORIES – AND THE SHAME OF WISHING MY MOTHER'S LIFE AWAY.

I remember my first Alzheimer's Association meeting the summer I moved my mother to be closer to me. I was given an information binder loaded with helpful tidbits on "all things dementia." Of everything in that binder, my eyes went straight to the chart that marked the progression of dementia by breaking it into three stages. I found myself re-reading Stages One and Two, comparing Mom's symptoms to each. As I read through the list of the particular behaviors associated with each stage, I remember very clearly thinking, *"Oh God, I hope she's more at Stage Two than One,"* and wondering how long it took to progress from one to the next.

That chart probably did more damage to me during my infant steps along my mother's path into dementia than her words did. It crushed me to read it. And yet I had been so hopeful when I found it in the binder. This was going to explain everything to me! All my questions were about to be answered! But they weren't. In fact, they created more questions. What does "more pronounced" mean? How long will she be doing this, or that? When will she get easier to be with? Will she ever be nice again? I needed a more specific timeline with more detailed examples. Just three stages seemed too generalized, and the part about this disease "sometimes lasting as long as 20 years" was beyond helpful – it was devastating.

Stages of Alzheimer's
Source: Alzheimer's Association

The symptoms of Alzheimer's disease worsen over time, although the rate at which the disease progresses varies. On average, a person with Alzheimer's lives four to eight years after diagnosis, but can live as long as 20 years, depending on other factors. Changes in the brain related to Alzheimer's begin years before any signs of the disease. This time period, which can last for years, is referred to as preclinical Alzheimer's disease.

The stages below provide an overall idea of how abilities change once symptoms appear and should only be used as a general guide. (Dementia is a general term to describe the symptoms of mental decline that accompany Alzheimer's and other brain diseases.)

The stages are separated into three categories: mild Alzheimer's disease, moderate Alzheimer's disease and severe Alzheimer's disease. Be aware that it may be difficult to place a person with Alzheimer's in a specific stage as stages may overlap.

Early-stage Alzheimer's (mild)
In the early stage of Alzheimer's, a person may function independently. He or she may still drive, work and be part of social activities. Despite this, the person may feel as if he or she is having memory lapses, such as forgetting familiar words or the location of everyday objects.

Symptoms may not be widely apparent at this stage, but family and close friends may take notice and a doctor would be able to identify symptoms using certain diagnostic tools.

Common difficulties include:

- Coming up with the right word or name.
- Remembering names when introduced to new people.
- Having difficulty performing tasks in social or work settings.
- Forgetting material that was just read.
- Losing or misplacing a valuable object.
- Experiencing increased trouble with planning or organizing.

During the early stage, it's possible for people with dementia to live well by taking control of their health and wellness and focusing their energy on aspects of their life that are most meaningful to them. In addition, this is the ideal time to put legal, financial and end-of-life plans in place because the person with dementia will be able to participate in decision-making.

Middle-stage Alzheimer's (moderate)

Middle-stage Alzheimer's is typically the longest stage and can last for many years. As the disease progresses, the person with Alzheimer's will require a greater level of care.

During the middle stage of Alzheimer's, the dementia symptoms are more pronounced. The person may confuse words, get frustrated or angry, and act in unexpected ways, such as refusing to bathe. Damage to nerve cells in the brain can also make it difficult for the person to express thoughts and perform routine tasks without assistance.

Symptoms, which vary from person to person, may include:

- Being forgetful of events or personal history.
- Being unable to recall information about themselves like their address or telephone number, and the high school or college they attended.
- Experiencing confusion about where they are or what day it is.
- Requiring help choosing proper clothing for the season or the occasion.
- Having trouble controlling their bladder and bowels.
- Experiencing changes in sleep patterns, such as sleeping during the day and becoming restless at night.
- Showing an increased tendency to wander and become lost.
- Demonstrating personality and behavioral changes, including suspiciousness and delusions or compulsive, repetitive behavior like hand-wringing or tissue shredding.

In the middle stage, the person living with Alzheimer's can still participate in daily activities with assistance. It's important to find out what the person can still do or find ways to simplify tasks. As the need for more intensive care increases, caregivers may want to consider respite care or an adult day center so they can have a temporary break from caregiving while the person living with Alzheimer's continues to receive care in a safe environment.

Late-stage Alzheimer's (severe)
In the final stage of the disease, dementia symptoms are severe. Individuals lose the ability to respond to their environment, to carry on a conversation and, eventually, to control movement. They may still say words or phrases, but communicating pain becomes difficult. As memory and cognitive skills continue to worsen, significant personality changes may take place and individuals need extensive care.

At this stage, individuals may:

- Require around-the-clock assistance with daily personal care.
- Lose awareness of recent experiences as well as of their surroundings.
- Experience changes in physical abilities, including walking, sitting and, eventually, swallowing.
- Have difficulty communicating.
- Become vulnerable to infections, especially pneumonia.

The person living with Alzheimer's may not be able to initiate engagement as much during the late stage, but he or she can still benefit from interaction in ways that are appropriate, like listening to relaxing music or receiving reassurance through gentle touch. During this stage, caregivers may want to use support services, such as hospice care, which focus on providing comfort and dignity at the end of life. Hospice can be of great benefit to people in the final stages of Alzheimer's and other dementias and their families.

How long does each stage of dementia Last?
Source: Reference.com

The stages of dementia can vary depending on the individual and the root causes of the dementia, notes Mayo Clinic. On average, people live about 4.5 years after being diagnosed with dementia, reports WebMD.

Alzheimer's disease often progresses in a more steady way that can make it difficult to identify the exact stages, states the Alzheimer Society of Ireland. Vascular dementia, another common type of dementia caused by small strokes that affect the brain's ability to function, often has more clear indications between the stages. This is because the decline generally only happens after another stroke occurs. Lewy Body dementia can be even more difficult to determine because the patient's abilities often change drastically from day to day. This type of dementia often lasts for six to 12 years before death occurs.

Alzheimer's disease can be more predictable, but it still varies wildly depending on the individual circumstances, explains HelpGuide.org. Stage one, or mild cognitive impairment, may last two to four years. Moderate Alzheimer's often lasts two to 10 years, while the third and most severe stage lasts one to three years or more. Alzheimer's disease also has a preclinical phase, in which the brain changes but there are no noticeable symptoms. This stage can last as long as 20 years, according to Mayo Clinic.

So there it was. Stage One: two to four years. Stage Two: two to ten years. And Stage Three: one to three years more, making that a grand total of five to seventeen years if you don't factor in that sneaky preclinical phase that I'm positive my mother had, beginning with my dad's death in 2000.

Not only were my hopes dashed to find that she was mostly only in Stage One, but the number of years I could expect to remain in this Hell were overwhelmingly ambiguous.

This was beyond unacceptable. I had to find more answers. I searched the internet and found that there was a similarly defined schedule of stages out there – seven to be exact. I tore through this new information, devouring its smaller, more specific transitions, searching for a match with my mother. Seven stages made the progression seem to move along more quickly, and it made it easier for me to track her from one stage to the next.

According to this new chart, Mom's behaviors fit somewhere between stage three and four, placing her further along on the scale and somehow providing me with the relief that this nightmare might be over sooner than I had initially believed.

My head swam as I realized I was wishing my mother's life away, and that it couldn't go fast enough for me. Did this happen to others as they read through the stages? I had no earthly idea. Did I admit this to anyone? Heck no! I wore my disgrace like a heavy wet coat every day. I woke up under the weight of it most mornings and fell asleep trapped inside it most nights.

No matter which set of stages you choose to align with, the unfathomably sad reality is that dementia is a slow-moving death sentence that will attempt to take down everyone within range. No one path is the same, but they're all similar enough to arrange into quantifiable stages. And when you think you've identified your loved one's stage, try to be patient, loving, and hold on to your hat.

Global Deterioration Scale for Assessment of Primary Degenerative Dementia
(The Seven Stages of Dementia)
Barry Reisberg, Clinical Director of the NY University School of Medicine's Silberstein Dementia Research Center

"One of the most difficult things to hear about dementia is that, in most cases, dementia is irreversible and incurable. However, with an early diagnosis and proper care, the progression of some forms of dementia can be managed and slowed down. The cognitive decline that accompanies dementia conditions does not happen all at once – the progression of dementia can be divided into seven distinct, identifiable stages.

Learning about the stages of dementia can help with identifying signs and symptoms early on, as well as assisting sufferers and caretakers in knowing what to expect in further stages. The earlier dementia is diagnosed, the sooner treatment can start."

Stage 1: No Cognitive Decline
Stage 1 of dementia can also be classified as the normal functioning stage. At this stage of dementia development, a patient generally does not exhibit any significant problems with memory, or any cognitive impairment. Stages 1-3 of dementia progression are generally known as "pre-dementia" stages.

Stage 2: Age Associated Memory Impairment
This stage features occasional lapses of memory most frequently seen in:

- Forgetting where one has placed an object
- Forgetting names that were once very familiar

Oftentimes, this mild decline in memory is merely normal age-related cognitive decline, but it can also be one of the earliest signs of degenerative dementia. At this stage, signs are still virtually undetectable through clinical testing. Concern for early onset of dementia should arise with respect to other symptoms.

Stage 3: Mild Cognitive Impairment
Clear cognitive problems begin to manifest in stage 3. A few signs of stage 3 dementia include:

- Getting lost easily
- Noticeably poor performance at work
- Forgetting the names of family members and close friends
- Losing or misplacing important objects
- Difficulty concentrating

Patients often start to experience mild to moderate anxiety as these symptoms increasingly interfere with day-to-day life. Patients who may be in this stage of dementia are encouraged to have a clinical interview with a clinician for proper diagnosis.

Stage 4: Mild Dementia
At this stage, individuals may start to become socially withdrawn and show changes in personality and mood. Denial of symptoms as a defense mechanism is commonly seen in stage 4. Behaviors to look for include:

- Decreased knowledge of current and/or recent events
- Difficulty remembering things about one's personal history
- Decreased ability to handle finances, arrange travel plans, etc.
- Disorientation

Difficulty recognizing faces and people in stage 4 dementia; individuals have no trouble recognizing familiar faces or traveling to familiar locations. However, patients in this stage will often avoid challenging situations in order to hide symptoms or prevent stress or anxiety.

Stage 5: Moderate Dementia
Patients in stage 5 need some assistance in order to carry out their daily lives. The main sign for stage 5 dementia is the inability to remember major details such as the name of a close family member or a home address. Patients may become disoriented about the time and place, have trouble making decisions, and forget basic information about themselves, such as a telephone number or address.

While moderate dementia can interfere with basic functioning, patients at this stage do not need assistance with basic functions such as using the bathroom or eating. Patients also still have the ability to remember their own names and generally the names of spouses and children.

Stage 6: Moderately Severe Dementia
When the patient begins to forget the names of their children, spouse, or primary caregivers, they are most likely entering stage 6 of dementia and will need full time care. In the sixth stage, patients are generally unaware of their surroundings, cannot recall recent

events, and have skewed memories of their personal past. Caregivers and loved ones should watch for:

- Delusional behavior
- Obsessive behavior and symptoms
- Anxiety, aggression, and agitation
- Loss of willpower

Patients may begin to wander, have difficulty sleeping, and in some cases will experience hallucinations.

Stage 7: Severe Dementia

Along with the loss of motor skills, patients will progressively lose the ability to speak during the course of stage 7 dementia. In the final stage, the brain seems to lose its connection with the body. Severe dementia frequently entails the loss of all verbal and speech abilities. Loved ones and caregivers will need to help the individual with walking, eating, and using the bathroom.

By identifying the earliest stages of dementia as they occur, you may be able to seek medical treatment quickly and delay the onset of later stages. Though most cases of dementia are progressive, some may be reversible, and sometimes dementia-like conditions may be caused by treatable underlying deficiencies or illnesses. The more aware you are of these stages, the quicker you will be able to react and seek help, either for yourself or for a loved one.

Those were the days when each new experience with my mother felt catastrophic, and I couldn't seem to keep up. When you're deep in it, it doesn't matter who tells you or how many times you hear, *"Don't be so hard on yourself, take a break, you're going to crash if you don't ease up."* You just wake up each morning, it's quiet for a moment, and then you remember this new life you're living. A creeping sense of wariness and even dread burrows itself deep in your stomach as you begin to execute your day, certain something terrible is about to happen.

And even when you've had one decent day, your loved

one's disease can manage to rattle you in ways you didn't think possible. Whether it was some mean spirited comment they delivered off-handedly or a voiced opinion so out of character for them it's repulsive to you. *"If my butt ever gets that big,"* said by Fay in front of an unsuspecting caregiver, *"just take me to the bridge and push me off."* I got better at separating my inner distaste from my outward reaction and learned to appear "unaffected" by my mother's bad behavior, but it didn't change the way I felt about her when it was happening. I didn't like anything about her at that moment and I wanted to leave her there – wherever that was.

It's taken me years to finally forgive myself for the shame of knowing full well the disgust I felt toward her during those times, even when I was able to control my responses toward her and show her at least patience.

> **To:** Carolyn
> **From:** Denise
>
> You're not going to believe where SAL-in-the-box was found today. In TCRP's kitchen. In the REFRIG-ERATOR AGAIN. What is it with her and the refrigerator?! And how did she get him in there undetected??!! There's almost always someone in there, but I guess the key word is "almost." The poor kitchen lady who found him! The only reason they knew it was Fay's SAL was because when she brought him to the Administration office to ask who he belonged to, one of the staff recognized him from your mom's room.

Years have passed and Fay is still with us as I write this part of the book, and about as healthy as any of us with a little age on. She recognizes me less than half the time now, and I just smile and tell her how nice she looks today and who did her nails? We'll wander over to the coffee counter and pour ourselves the first of several cups we'll have during my visit, thank goodness for decaf. We'll admire Dolly, and I'll ask if she had breakfast, and she'll always respond with her perfunctory, "No." Whether she's referring to Dolly or to herself, it doesn't matter, and I don't ask. We'll walk past the courtyard windows, and I'll comment on the flowers and a bird, if we're lucky. On her foggier days she'll likely ask me if I'm that woman she saw in the magazine and I'll smile an agreeable, "Yes." She struggles for words these days, and I find myself filling in the blanks as she bobs her head, "Yes," when I guess correctly.

She wears Depends full-time now, no longer nights only, and I'm reminded of the times she used to make comments about another resident at The Community Resting Place who wore them. Steel-jawed, she'd recite her favorite mantra, "Just take me to the bridge..." I wonder how she processes in her mind the fact that she wears them now, but I suppose I already know the answer. That memory is long gone for her, and she doesn't give it a second thought as she allows some caregiver to help her on with hers each day.

She's softer and smaller now, like she's lost three inches from her frame. She moves much more carefully, and I find myself with my hand at her back or my arm linked in hers as we navigate the hallways. She doesn't seem to mind like she once did, insisting "I can walk by myself," or "You don't have to slow down for me." Her spirit has quieted, and it's as much a heartbreak as it is a relief to me now. Just another conflict I've learned to live with.

I find it so interesting that when I'm engaged in conversation with someone about my mother and her dementia, they often follow with, "Oh, that's too bad. Is it Alzheimer's?" I don't know, is it? Is their need to label it their way of connecting with me on some common level? And maybe by doing so, they're able to say, "Oh yes, I've heard of Alzheimer's. I know what you're going through."

The fact is, she's never received an official diagnosis. We

couldn't get her to comply during any of her exams. As soon as she realized what was going on she'd go silent, and when pushed with each additional question, she'd finally respond shrilly, "I know what you're trying to do! I'm not crazy! And I'm not answering any of your silly questions." Exam over.

Dementia is dementia, as far as my mother is concerned. I understand there are differing nuances among the types, but it doesn't matter much to me which kind she has. Whether her behaviors resemble someone with Alzheimer's, Lewy Body Disease, Frontal Lobe, or Vascular Dementia, I don't feel the need to know anymore, and I don't need to distress her any further to find out. She's confused, she's often unsettled, and she's very suspicious (wouldn't you be if you woke up in the morning and nothing looked the same as you left it?). That's enough for me to know and more than enough for me to manage.

These last several years with Fay have granted me an extensive study into internal conflict, and I feel like I've come out the other side with my diploma. I've learned that the inner struggle is pretty much always there; it's just magnified when one is pushed to one's limits. And I've learned I need to simply notice my bad feelings instead of desperately try to extinguish them, to not give them any more power than my good feelings. I believe we all have the angel and the devil on our shoulders, and they chatter constantly, sometimes one louder than the other, and always more so when we're under siege.

My hope is that you'll say, "Aha!" here and there through my story, and you'll connect with some random incident or two that will make you feel a little more "normal." Or you'll recognize someone going through something similar in this story who's suffering and share this with them. I still remember telling my doctor that I was convinced something was seriously wrong with me, that I shouldn't be having the feelings I was having or responding to things in the manner I was. I can look back at it all now and laugh. I mean, really laugh. There are so many stories here that bring a chuckle to me now, but at the time reduced me to tears. I used to worry that my mother was gone to me forever, and that this newer, meaner version was dumped onto my lap as my new, unwelcome responsibility.

I know now that I was wrong. She's still my mom. She's still somewhere inside that poor little peanut head. Confused, but a little more peaceful, finally. They told me it would get easier...

I don't know how our story ends, hers and mine, because as of right now, it continues. Will I have to move her again? Will she be one of the ones who lingers, losing her ability to swallow and focus? Will I have to make the decision for life support? Or will she fall and break a hip, then develop pneumonia like the stories we all hear? These are the cruel realities of this insidious, heartless disease that will choose someone like my wonderful, loving mother to hound until her death.

It's a discussion I have these days. Which is worse? To lose your mind and still have a strong, healthy body, or to keep your wits and witness your body's slow and eventual decline? Sam's 90-year-old mother has been living with him these past few years after suffering a stroke during one of her summer visits. It's heart wrenching to listen to her describe the indignities she's suffered from her body letting her down, fully aware and deeply regretful of all the things she's lost. My mother, now 85, thinks she's working at her old job in the hospital when I was 14 and happily picks up the broom to sweep a speck into the corner or adjusts someone's napkin around their neck for them. It's a tough call, very individual, and probably impossible to decide – and we don't get to choose anyway.

To: Carolyn
From: Ginny

We went to visit Sam's Mom at the hospital across the street – this time Fay was game for it (I never know). She seems to be such a comfort for Hannah, and Hannah seems to adore Fay. Fay usually is very lucid around her, saying all appropriate and supporting things while holding Hannah's hand. Very sweet. Hannah said that Sam had been there this morning, with his own spinach & potatoes that he cooked for her. The only subject that Fay got tripped up on was where she lives at present. When I pointed out the proximity of TCRP and Hannah asked Fay directly if she lived there, Fay replied "No!"

"Where *do* you live?" Hannah asked, and Fay answered, "I live at home!" Where exactly that is... remains a question mark.

When we got back to TCRP, we finished up our 300-pc quilt puzzle. In the middle Fay kept asking her usual "What did I have for breakfast? I don't remember... I didn't have breakfast!" and I told her if she were hungry, she could always ask the kitchen for snacks. She went and I could hear the conversation. They were very accommodating, and I could tell this wasn't the first time they encountered this scenario with Fay. She came back to the puzzle with a big grin and a WHOLE corned beef sandwich wrapped up in a napkin (wonder where her weight gain is coming from??). Fay immediately gave me half and required that I eat it, despite my saying I wasn't that hungry. Dilemma – eat it and make Fay happy and look like a mooch to staff, or not eat it and be badgered to do so by Fay for the next 15 minutes. I'm thinking of making a financial donation at the end of each month to them for the assorted extra coffees and such.

So we continue to walk with Fay. Now it's just from her room to the dining room. And she enjoys it. And she doesn't remember that she used to walk for miles or that she once climbed cherry trees. And everything is just the way that it is.

$\mathcal{F}$AY'S NEXT MOVE.

Everything was changing again. Even my calls from TCRP were different. They were no longer information sharing calls seeking my input on how to tackle Fay's new behavior. Now they mostly began with, *"We have a problem. Your mother is wandering into other residents' rooms at night and peeing on their floor."* Or *"We have a problem. Your mother is roaming from table to table during dinner and sampling the food off other residents' plates and she's upsetting them."* Or *"We have a problem. Your mother is slipping into residents' rooms and helping herself to their things. We've had three complaints from their families today."*

These were usually lengthy conversations that included questions from me on whether they were using the basket of folding towels to keep her busy, or was she being invited to sweep the floors in the dining room – both schemes that had worked wonders over at Serenity Home and were good for my busy little bee. The honest answer was no, they were not.

I was politely reminded that The Community Resting Place was an assisted living facility, and that was the scope of their training, staff-to-resident ratio, and responsibility. It was a place where an elderly person could live in their own private quarters and not have to worry about fixing their meals or doing their laundry. There were activities to entertain residents, but it was not staff's job to monitor and direct them all day. There simply weren't enough of them to do that, along with their other duties. The place for that was across the street at the Advanced Care Wing located in the north end of the hospital. Everyone referred to it as the ACW and assumed the same knowing expression when they did.

"Holy Heaven, Mom can't be ready for that place," was all I could think as I listened to the manager at TCRP tell me exactly that. Here we were again, facing move number four.

My vision of the Advanced Care Wing was of old people strapped into chairs or lying in bed, as white as their sheets. A place like that couldn't be the right fit for my mother yet, and how was she going to adjust to this new, constrictive environment? I honestly didn't know how this move was going to work, but I was being pushed in that direction by The Community Resting Place.

The first thing I did was make a call to the Advanced Care Wing to speak with the manager, Darla, a lovely and encouraging woman who invited me to come meet her and tour the facility, so I did the next day. I was amazed that it wasn't as asylum-bright or hospital-sterile as I had imagined. Some of the residents were surprisingly mobile and alert, sprinkled about the facility. I noticed several of them either reading, listening to music, or watching TV in the main room. Their dining room was just like TCRP's, and overall it wasn't the depressing institution I had expected.

We wrapped up the tour back at Darla's office where she carefully explained the difference between assisted living care and extended care. It looked like my mother would be well taken care of there. She ran through the many ways they were trained and capable to handle the stages that people with dementia inevitably move through. The cost for care was significantly higher, and I thought I was going to throw up on her desk when she told me the monthly fee schedule was going to be over $7k. There was no way I was going to be able to afford that without selling a piece of property, which was my personal source of income. *"Unless,"* she offered, *"your mother qualifies for Medicaid,"* which she did, just a few months prior. She reassured me that she would make the appropriate calls and confirm my mother's coverage would kick in once her Social Security and pension income were used to pay for the bulk of the expenses. I didn't care what they took; they could have it all.

The next step was for Darla and Cathy, the patient coordinator, to go across the street and meet my mother for an "Assessment of Compatibility" interview with their facility. Oh no, another exam Fay was sure to fail. I wanted so badly to coach them on the best way to handle her, *"Don't ask her what year this is! Or who's the President. Or the names of her children!"*

But it was Denise who reminded me that they were the professionals, and they did this sort of thing every day. *"Let them do their job."* Well, they didn't exactly do this sort of thing *every day with Fay.* I knew how my mother could respond whenever she felt scrutinized or judged. *"Let them do their job, Carolyn."* All I could do was hope for a good day on Mom's part, and meaningless-sounding conversation on theirs.

I found out later that they opened their interview with, *"Do you know what year it is?"* and *"Do you know the name of our new President?"* Shit. Then they explained to my mother that they were there to *"assess her in order to move her over to the Advanced Care Wing so that they could take better care of her needs, and what did she think of that?"* Shit again. Turns out they had a generally lovely visit even after that, according to Denise, who hovered quietly nearby.

Denise also admitted that my mother ended the interview with, *"That all sounds like a very nice idea, but don't count on it."*

Everything came to a grinding halt after that. I didn't know if it was due to room availability, staff-to-resident ratio that needed to be beefed up, or that Mom had scared them into reconsidering, but Robert and I had already left on our annual trip to Florida, and I wasn't about to call the ACW to ask about the delay in Mom's transfer and get started on the wrong foot with them. In my mind, my mother was safely tucked away at The Community Resting Place, albeit always in trouble and a pain in the butt for them, but I was letting nature take its course on this one.

I continued to receive increasingly unhappy-sounding calls from TCRP, with comments like, *"We don't understand; we sent her paperwork over to them months ago and they keep dragging their feet."* I would remain as quiet and calm on the phone as I could, offer my assistance if they needed me to make a call (please-oh-please don't ask me to make a call), and thank them for keeping me informed.

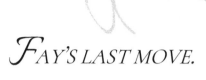

$\mathcal{F}$AY'S LAST MOVE.

Year Seven – Stage 6, some 7
(Moderately Severe Dementia/Severe Dementia)

Then one day a few months later still, Denise called me on a Friday afternoon, *"Did you get a call from the ACW? They're moving your mother on Monday."* I choked back panic, *"No one has called me! How am I going to arrange this so quickly from Florida?"* My next call was to Darla at the Advanced Care Wing, who told me she was just getting ready to call me about Monday's move. Fine, fine, but what did I need to do? *"Can she have all her clothes or just a certain amount, and what about her dresser? Should we leave her lamps behind? And can we hang her paintings?"*

> **To:** Carolyn
> **From:** Ginny
>
> It sounds like Monday is the day for Fay's next move! Denise called me because I told her I'd help when the time came. Denise is taking her to lunch while I hang Fay's paintings and make it look homey.
>
> As far as "the story" to tell this time, I was thinking of telling her that TCRP needs renovation work and that everyone had to be relocated temporarily (because of all the snow on the roof!), then we can embellish if necessary by telling her she got the best hotel room because she has seniority. I'll try to make several visits in the coming weeks so she has more company. I know Denise comes often; she's such a sweetheart in that way.

Denise and Ginny, complete with wings and halos, handled nearly every detail while I quarterbacked from Florida. Denise arranged for Jacob, The Community Resting Place's maintenance man, to help move one of Mom's dressers (no room for two) across the street and into her new room while Ginny took Mom for a walk. Ginny then turned her over to Denise for a "lunch date" while she put Mom's bed together and hung all her paintings. Then, Ginny scooted back over to TCRP to take Mom for another walk while Denise transferred all of Mom's clothes over to the ACW. Denise was waiting for Fay and Ginny in the living room after their second walk and the three of them ambled across the street to *"check out the new condos Denise had heard about."*

Those two were at it from before noon until 7:30 that night, settling Fay into her room, eating dinner together, and keeping her company. Robert swore they must both be atoning for some crime in a previous life to be the angels that they were to Fay (and me), and I concurred.

We made it one full day before the first call came in from the ACW. *"Your mother tried to leave via the hospital doors last night, and it took us all night to convince her to leave the doors alone."* Well duh, I could've warned them about that. It's her first night in a strange place, she can't sleep, and there's a set of closed doors leading to a hallway that could very well contain the Ark of the Covenant. A simple, *"Oh Fay! There you are! I have your cup of nice hot coffee right over here for you,"* would've done the trick. Instead, my caller told me they put a sign on the doors that said, "FAY, TURN AROUND."

"And how did that work?" I asked.

"Well... we're going to have a meeting tomorrow about what else we can do to keep her away from those doors."

The next few days were a blur of back-and-forth phone calls and a patient intake conference call with me on speaker phone to a roundtable of staff.

The first issue was, of course, the doors and Mom's fixation on them. We discussed various ways to distract her and help redirect her focus onto something else, like the discovery of a fresh pot of coffee or a beautiful vase of flowers at the front desk someone had just delivered.

She also wasn't eating. I described to them the way I was raised – with the polite, *"No, thank you,"* whenever we visited friends and I was offered something to eat or drink. My parents instilled in me a strong belief that I was never to inconvenience somebody by having them do work in order to serve me, and especially never to take food/ candy/drinks from anyone. As hard as it was for *me* to negotiate a healthy balance between my upbringing and something a little more socially acceptable as an adult, imagine the probability of my poor little mother changing her ways at this late date.

Ask my mom if she's hungry and she'll say, *"No, I just ate."* Would she like something to drink? *"No, thank you, I'm not thirsty."* She could be parched with a grumbling stomach that you could hear from the doorway, and she'd give you the same automatic response. I told them that she would eat almost anything they handed her, as long as they couched it with, *"Fay! Look what I found in the kitchen! They have extra!"* Or *"Fay! My mother just baked banana bread and brought me three loaves! I don't have room in my freezer for this one, want it?"*

Our conference call ended on a high note, with everyone feeling motivated to try out their newfound tactics on Fay. It was agreed that we would follow up in a few days with a progress report. I thanked everyone at the table, told them how much I appreciated them (I truly did), and hung up the phone as I released a blast of air I hadn't realized I'd been holding.

I can't remember if three days passed or four before receiving my follow-up call, but I DO remember my stomach dropping when I saw the number light up my phone. I knew the nature of the news was a 50/50 bet at best, and I hadn't seen favorable odds in a while. But the woman on the phone addressed me in a calm, friendly voice and began with, *"Hello Carolyn! This is the day nurse at the ACW, and we have positive news to report!"*

She told me that Mom's appetite was increasing, which was good, and they'd rolled a bookcase in front of the hospital doors so they'd be out of Mom's direct sight, which also seemed to help. What I DIDN'T expect to hear was that Mom's newest-and-repeated activity was to wander into residents' rooms and poop on their floors. Simply horrific. But even worse, she was wiping her hands on the floors and anywhere else she could reach to clean up.

The friendly day nurse assured me this wasn't deviant behavior and more so a symptom of her recent constipation and preoccupation with "getting it out." When the opportunity arose she merely took full advantage, and that often included finding the nearest room for privacy. The wiping on the floor and furniture was simply because she was helping it out with her hands and needed a place to wipe it off. When you broke it down like that, it made perfect sense in my mother's mind, regardless of what it did in mine.

They planned to incorporate more water into her daily routine and provide a laxative. She reiterated the necessity of keeping Mom out of residents' rooms and the safety risk it presented. I brought up the laundry-basket-of-towels-to-fold trick, and she seemed determined to try it. I wouldn't say we ended the call on as upbeat a note as the patient intake roundtable, but we did have a plan, and they hadn't told me she needed to leave. Yet.

A few weeks had gone by since those follow-up calls, and just as I was feeling like maybe we were out of the woods, my phone signaled an incoming call from the ACW one afternoon.

I took three breaths and answered, only to immediately be informed I was on speaker phone with the day nurse, office manager, and facility administrator. They got right down to business with an update on my mom's newest behavior: Helping residents disconnect their bed and wheelchair alarms. You know, the ones that discharge a shrill blast if you stand up from your chair or try to exit your bed unattended? Meant to keep you from falling and getting a concussion or breaking a hip? Yes, those.

Apparently, the residents who had them didn't like them, and no amount of pleading could convince a caregiver there to disconnect them – until they asked my mother. Fay was found happily darting from room to room, Nurse Nightingale, and assisting each resident with the removal of that pesky strap. Their very real fear was that she would take it upon herself to disconnect OTHER things, like IV drips, oxygen, or anything else with a tube.

I agreed that this was indeed an intolerable new habit of hers, but it was when the administrator cut in with, *"And I feel I must tell you that when I walked into my office this morning, your mother was sitting on my trash can, pooping into it,"* that I knew what was coming next, and it did. She'd been there just over one month, and I was verbally being issued my mother's 30-day exit notification. A dozen questions whirled around my brain, but the only one I managed to ask before hanging up was whether the administrator knew why my mother had pooped into her trash can, and she said that she did. Upon entering her office, she asked Fay exactly that, to which she replied, *"Because your door was open."*

They were lovely about it, really. They offered to help me locate a more appropriate facility with an even greater staff-to-resident ratio. As much as we all thought they could handle my mother's needs, the Advanced Care Wing in my town was more equipped to handle bed-ridden residents who were nearing the end of their lives. My perfectly ambulatory mother with a curiosity about everything and a healthy ability to satisfy it required more hands-on supervision than even they had predicted.

$\mathcal{F}$AY'S LAST, LAST MOVE.

Year Seven and Eight – Stage 7
(Severe Dementia)

Our answer came a few days later in the form of Rainbow Ranch Senior Living in Sandpoint, ID. And more specifically, the women's dementia wing called "The Carriage House." Situated in a quiet corner of the facility, this eight-bed wing was designed with my mother (and other mothers) in mind. The staff-to-resident ratio was high, and they didn't even flinch when I fessed up about her troublesome wandering and inappropriate pooping. After some lengthy telephone meetings and an overnighted package to Florida with forms to sign and notarize, my mother became the newest resident of Rainbow Ranch! It was amazingly easy and almost alarming that I could place my mother so quickly into the care of another facility from 3,000 miles away.

Denise, Ginny, and I were all disappointed that she was being moved 35 deer-dodging highway miles away, which would mean a decrease in her number of regular visits, but we came up with a plan to rotate our trips around each other so we would never be there on the same day.

Yet another new plan was devised to whisk Fay away to Sandpoint without upsetting her and without her seeing her clothes being packed. Enter again Denise and Ginny, fibbers extraordinaire. It was a simple ladies' lunch, *"with a few boxes of things Denise needed to drop at a friend's house."* They spent the afternoon eating lunch and exploring Mom's new digs, with Mom falling asleep in her new room right afterward. They decided to slip out while she dozed, instructing staff to call me if she awoke upset. She surprised all of us and slept through the night, waking up the next morning to toast and eggs.

There were the usual (at least by now they were usual to me) calls in the beginning with questions like, *"Does your mother like cereal?"* or *"Can your mother have anything she wants to eat? We're trying to put some weight on her."* Their main challenge was her rapid weight loss. She tended to stop eating each time she'd been moved, and she'd been moved twice in as many months. Staff worked on rebuilding her appetite by constantly enticing her with her favorite foods.

I returned home from Florida a few weeks after her move to Rainbow Ranch and made it my first stop on my drive home from the airport. I was required to sign in at the front desk, make the short trek through a maze of hallways and wheelchairs, and then press a four-digit code on a security pad that activated the swinging doors separating the Carriage House from the rest of the facility.

She looked frail, like a smaller, even older version of Fay. I hadn't seen her in three months, and the physical change was startling. She met my gaze, but her expression remained the same. There was no hint of recognition or happiness to see me. I pulled a chair closer to hers and sang, *"Hello MeeMaw!"* as I leaned in to kiss her forehead. She lurched backward to avoid my advance and brought her hand up to swat me. I'd forgotten how averse she was to affection, and my quick movements clearly frightened her.

I sat quietly next to her for thirty minutes. There was no conversation between us. She just rocked to and froe in her chair and hummed. A caregiver joined us and introduced herself, saying how much they enjoyed having Fay with them. I struggled to smile and thanked her. Frankly, I couldn't imagine how enjoyable Mom could be, but I was happy to hear something positive about her newest move.

Leaving her was easy. She kept her gaze fixed on the window as I carefully laid my hand on her shoulder to squeeze it goodbye. The difficult part was the backward trail I should've memorized to return to the reception area.

By the time I reached the front desk, I'd been tugged at, pulled on, and screeched at by the myriad residents in wheelchairs parked in the hallways. I signed out, let myself in my truck, and leaned over the steering wheel sobbing.

My mother was a shell. She was locked away in a confined area of what felt like an insane asylum, and I was the one who put her there. Again. It didn't matter that I'd arranged safe shelter for her with more intensive care when she needed it – all I could see were my mistakes, and this one was just another decision I'd made that felt wrong after I'd made it.

I was always one step behind with her, playing catch-up to meet her ever-progressing needs, and it never felt like enough. Like placing Band-Aids on a gaping axe cut, her dementia's progression was a speeding train, and I was running on foot.

By the time I returned home I'd replayed the entire visit several times in my head. I chided myself for my melodrama and repeated all of the positive things now happening for my mother and me. The facility was actually perfect. She was surrounded by caregivers in a wing designated for memory care. And they were happy to have her.

To: Denise
From: Carolyn

I'm baaaack!!! First stop: Mom. Oh my gosh it was so sad. She didn't really look at me, and she's so tiny! They said they're trying to fatten her up with anything she likes and handle her insulin levels accordingly. I counted four caregivers in just her wing!

I began driving to Sandpoint every week, turning it into a day of errands after visiting my mother. Most times I dropped in to find her seated in an overstuffed chair with a tray table in front of her, filled with any combination of grilled cheese sandwiches, green beans, biscuits, or mashed potatoes.

The grilled cheese sandwiches were hit and miss, but I quickly discovered that she now loved any kind of pastry. We didn't have many when I was growing up, and she always preferred fruit over processed sweets, but this was the ever-evolving Fay, and I was constantly reminded that anything was possible with her now. So I went on the hunt for a cookie that wouldn't aggravate her insulin levels. My neighbor, also a diabetic, turned me on to our local Safeway's "Fruit Bars" from the bakery department. They were a lackluster combination of whole wheat flour and raisins, but when those bars came out, so did a huge grin and renewed enthusiasm to eat. Within three months Mom put six pounds back onto her pitifully shrinking frame. Her move from The Community Resting Place to ACW to Rainbow Ranch had cost her eleven.

Meals at a senior living facility are a daily highlight and met with anticipation and excitement (at least in each of the four my mother lived). Residents who could walk were often found loitering or pacing right outside the dining area before the allotted time. Even those in wheelchairs would park nearby so they could quickly snag their assigned seat, *"before anyone else took it."* They never seemed to catch on that their table placement was prearranged, as was everyone else's. So with each resident aiming for their favorite spot at the table, the risk of a seat being stolen was eliminated.

Mom had been no different. She always found a reason to be near the dining room just before mealtime. But these days her focus on eating had waned and it took a herculean effort to get her to clean her plate. It was like watching a two-year-old eat. If left to her own devices, she'd invariably pour her apple juice into her bowl of steamed carrots and stab holes through them with her straw. Some days I'd find her at the lunch table with mashed potatoes in her coffee. I could practically catch the daggers she shot at me with her eyes when I told her not to do that, but she never uttered a word; she just sat there, pinch-faced.

If I plucked a carrot out of the bowl and waved it at her exclaiming, *"Look! Carrots!"* she'd take a bite. And then it would start all over again with her jamming meatloaf into her pudding. Mealtime with Fay took a full hour of the caregivers' constant focus, and the dining room usually had twice as many residents as staff.

I don't know how they managed to cover an entire room

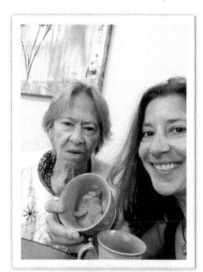

~ *"I don't know how those got there!"* ~

and ensure each person consumed their meal reasonably well. I DO know that by showing up at mealtime, I often encouraged my mother to take a few extra bites, something I'd strongly urge anyone to do when visiting their loved one. You'll make certain they get a little more to eat (so important to their health at this stage) and it'll give you something loving to do with them.

Rainbow Ranch was different from her last three homes. It was specially focused, complete with more caregivers per resident. The place was teeming with scrubs-wearing smiling faces, and The Carriage House wing always had an engaged group of them in constant motion. I no longer felt like I had to entertain everyone, since they were usually quite occupied when I arrived.

My visits were always at random times, since it was hard

to pick one set day or time until I could see what the week ahead looked like. I was always pleased (and relieved) with the "condition" in which I found my mother each time. We've all heard the nursing home horror stories about abuse, neglect, and general uncleanliness; and frankly, all my eggs were in this home's basket. I couldn't afford to find much wrong with the way they treated my mother because I had no place else for her to go. But she was always dressed nicely, with her shoes on and her hair (bless it) at least washed and combed. If she didn't have Dolly in her lap, she had the purring toy kitty, or an activity board designed for toddlers that entertained her for hours.

Her favorite was the "latches activity board," by toy makers Melissa and Doug (designed for 2+ year olds), with every type of handle, hook, and latch attached to different doors that swung open to expose a cute dog, horse, or pirate's chest of jewels. She never could figure out how to unlatch any of them and was both startled and delighted every time I opened one to show her there was something behind it. When I stopped, she'd pick right back up again, rattling and wiggling the latches unsuccessfully for hours.

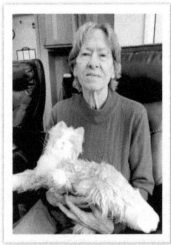
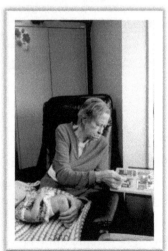

~ *Well-loved kitty* ~   ~ *Two-timing Dolly &*
activity board ~

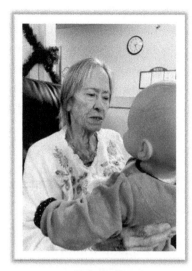

~ Ugly Dolly ~

Dolly and Kitty were always out on rotation for varying degrees of sanitizing. Mom's favorite thing to do was feed them – any sort of food went into any possible orifice. Poor Kitty's face, ears, and butthole were constantly caked with peaches and pudding, and stained red from Mom's juice. Ditto for Dolly.

I arrived one day to find Mom with a huge baby doll (naked of course, since everyone got a stripping under her care), with an oversized head, square bean bag body, and stiff plastic appendages that stuck straight out unnaturally. Its eyes stared forward and were perpetually open, and its hair was painted directly onto its scalp. This was *not* her lovely, lifelike Dolly. In fact, it was so oversized and odd looking that we named it Ugly Dolly. It was unsettling to watch her interact with it, sometimes shaking it aggressively and other times cradling it lovingly.

I asked a caregiver where Dolly was and she replied, *"Hmm... haven't seen her in a while. This one is Fay's new favorite."* And it was – for months and months. Dolly was MIA and Ugly Dolly had claimed its place on my mother's lap. Kind of like the child who prefers pots and pans over toys, my mother proved that all my trouble and expense to bring her Dolly was for naught.

So many visits over the next year brought new and unexpected experiences with Fay. She was 87 now and had lived longer than any of her siblings or her mother. One sunny afternoon I decided to take a quick drive to Sandpoint and

211

treat myself to a Starbucks while I was there. It was after lunchtime, and as I made my way down the main hallway to The Carriage House I walked right past Fay using a walker and flanked by two smiling caregivers. I spun around and said, *"Well, hello Zippy!"* and she beamed at me, flashing a huge, toothless grin. I grabbed my phone and snapped a photo that captured a woman with a face filled with complete joy. Time may have been progressing, but Fay was still walking.

The Carriage House was always bustling with activity and staff were kept busy. Each resident there had her own personality and particular needs, Mom's roommate Joan was

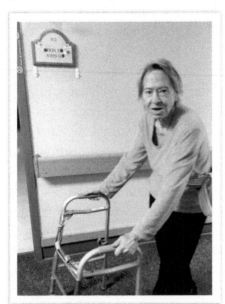

~ Grinning like she'd just gotten away with something ~

convinced she needed to help with some large gathering and was constantly stealing napkins and paper cups for her big event. She could be found busily rearranging table settings and fussing about the time and who was going to show up, and when. She was a handful to keep away from the other residents' plates during meal-time. Another resident, Helen, just knew she'd been accidently left behind by her family and her daughter was desperately trying to reach her but couldn't find the place. I was given the same interrogation each time I passed her chair as I entered the main living room to visit with Mom.

"Did you run into my daughter out front?"

– I'm sorry Helen, I didn't.

"She was supposed to be here hours ago."

– I'm sure she'll be here any minute.

"I think she's been in an accident/can't find the place/is driving in circles..."

– She'll be fine; how about a cup of coffee while we wait?

"Oh, what a nice idea."

Margaret declared she had starred in whichever movie was playing on the large screen TV and remembered the set design well. It distressed her when her claims failed to illicit the proper response of admiration from the five or six residents seated in the living room with her.

The common theme I noticed among the residents during my visits was the constant low- to high-grade distress level they all seemed to be on the verge of. Each of them needed some degree of reassurance, cajoling, and diversion on a regular basis. Staff were constantly playing games, singing songs, and generally distracting them, but their anxious stories seemed to play on repeating loops. Very few happy, contented dementia patients ever crossed my path. I imagined an eight-hour shift had to feel twice as long for those caregivers. At least it would for me.

Our routine is the same now. I greet her with a kiss on the cheek and she flinches away from me, hand flying up at me. Then her face opens into a smile, and I think maybe she knows me, but she doesn't say my name anymore. She doesn't speak, other than to parrot back a "hello" or "goodbye." She points. Things on the floor bother her. The shiny levers on the reclining chairs plague her as she tries incessantly to reach them. She doesn't like the lamp cords plugged into the outlets and begs to pull them out. Luckily, Mom can't even lean forward to get out of her chair without an aide asking, "Where are you going, Fay?" No more pooping in residents' rooms, taking food off her neighbor's plate, or disconnecting bed alarms for her new friends. I bring magazines and we flip through the pages together. She no longer points to a dog and says, "dog," or a recipe and says, "I'd like that."

Now I do the pointing. Anything I comment on is noted by a nod of the head. I'll ask her if she'd ever wear a crazy outfit like the one on the magazine cover and she'll laugh and laugh. I bring my ukulele now and play the few songs I know by heart. "The Lion Sleeps Tonight" is only semi-enthusiastically received, but I nail it with Johnny Cash's "Do Lord." Every lady knows the words, including, somehow, my mother, so I play it over and over until she hisses at me to stop. This woman who can't form complete sentences and won't say my name can somehow still sing all the verses to almost any gospel song.

According to Petr Janata, a cognitive neuroscientist at University of California, Davis, it's quite normal for dementia patients to remember songs even when they can't remember what they had for lunch. "The fact that **the prefrontal cortex** is among the last of the brain regions to atrophy may explain the ability of patients with Alzheimer's who have severe memory loss to remember songs from their distant past" (Jeremy Hsu, LiveScience.com 2009).

My trips to Sandpoint have developed into a comfortable routine now. In the past, before my mom was moved to Rainbow Ranch, it was a drive I'd make maybe once a month – my Home Depot run and Starbucks treat. Now it's on my weekly calendar. I had a tough time squeezing in a day each week at first, but now it's something I look forward to. I'll typically spend an hour visiting with my mother, get a lovely bowl of soup for lunch at Winter Ridge Market, followed by a leisurely browse through Home Depot. I'll head home with a hot Americano and the stereo turned off. It's become my peaceful time to replay the visit in my head and reflect on our interaction that day.

I'll admit that I usually cry a little of the way home. It's no longer about my hurt feelings over something she said to me, *since she no longer speaks, but more over her decline. It's so pronounced now that it's impossible for me to leave our visits any way but incredibly sad.*

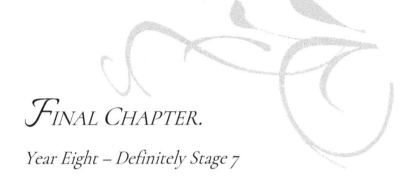

*F*INAL CHAPTER.

Year Eight – Definitely Stage 7

I was back in Florida enjoying the last part of my winter stay while the rest of north Idaho dreamt of spring. My phone played the wind chime tone, signaling a call from Rainbow Ranch. I shifted into alarm mode when I realized it was only 7am in Idaho – an early shift call.

"Hi Carolyn, this is Sharon from Rainbow Ranch." She didn't follow with the usual, *"There's nothing wrong, we're just calling to let you know..."* This time, her call was to inform me that my mother had woken up this morning without the use of her left side.

The morning caregiver noticed Mom's inability to help get herself dressed and called a nurse in to assess her. They noticed immediately that the left side of her face sagged and paged the on-call doctor. The good news was that she was alert, and they were able to sit her up in her chair in the living area. But she wasn't making her usual "chirps." She'd long stopped using her words, but she'd make these little bird-like noises that everyone was familiar with as her way of communicating, and this morning she was silent.

The date was Monday, March 23, 2020, and we as a nation were just beginning to grasp the fact that we were moving in the direction of a pandemic.

This new turn of events spurred me into changing my already scheduled April 7 Tampa/Spokane flight. I was ready to return home to Idaho anyway, so I'd just leave a little sooner. What I didn't anticipate was the extent to which the Covid-19 outbreak was about to affect airline travel. This was the end of March, and the Coronavirus was already reaching epic proportions in the United States. Interstate travel was just beginning to become affected. I was able to change my flight home to early Friday morning, March 27, only four more days to wait. I had just enough time to button up my house and make arrangements with Denise to pick me up at the airport. That alone was a pretty big favor to ask anyone, considering the drive to Spokane International Airport was a five-hour round trip.

By Thursday, March 26, the United States reportedly led the world in confirmed Covid-19 cases. It seemed like every day delivered alarming new statistics about this sudden and mysterious virus. I couldn't have predicted that the CDC was about to issue a travel advisory, starting with New York, New Jersey, and Connecticut, effective March 28. I'd booked my flight just days before the stay-at-home directive had been issued for Idaho, with many states following suit, including Florida on April 3. I was riding the crest of this Coronavirus tsunami and didn't even realize it yet.

On Thursday the 26th, the on-call nurse phoned to report that Mom was no longer able to sit up, that she hadn't eaten much dinner last night and was still in bed today, sleeping. They'd called in a speech therapist to assess her ability to swallow, and she didn't appear to be in pain. About that time, I received my first text from the airlines that my morning flight on Friday had been moved to the afternoon. I called Denise to give her my new arrival time. She told me not to worry about it, but we were both a little apprehensive about driving home from the airport in the dark.

One thing about that trip is that a copilot is always welcomed. Their job is to spot deer and elk along the highway; but at night, it's even more necessary, and more than a little nerve-wracking. Neither of us considered the flight delay to be anything beyond a shuffling of planes due to the heavy demand of passengers flying to their random destinations due to this flu. It was an inconvenience to our planned daytime drive home from the airport, but we didn't give it anymore thought than that.

At 3am Friday morning, my phone pinged a message from the airline that my rescheduled afternoon flight had been canceled and moved to Saturday morning. I waited until 9am to text Denise (who was relieved not to have to drive in the dark) and Robert (who was aggravated that these cancellations were still coming).

He called me right back to ask for my confirmation number, and all I could think was, *"Please don't get involved, this is all under control and I'm flying out on Saturday morning anyhow."*

An hour later, I received a text from him saying, *"Stay off the phone, you're about to get a call from the airline."* No call came, so an hour later I called him. Apparently, he'd finally gotten through to the airlines, and while trying to upgrade me to a surprise first class seat on my Saturday morning flight, he was told that THAT flight had also just been canceled, and that there wouldn't be another option flying from Tampa to Spokane until the following Tuesday (April 7, my original flight).

After demanding to speak with a supervisor, he was put through to Terrell, with whom he went round and round over the fact that he was not Carolyn Testa, and how could Terrell schedule anything for a customer who wasn't present to confirm the terms? I'll never know the rest of that conversation, but suffice it to say a call came in from an Atlanta number and Terrell was on the other end, thanking me for being a valued customer of Delta Airlines (I was?) and reassuring me that he'd moved me to a different flight for

Saturday afternoon connecting through Minneapolis. His last words, after thanking me again were, *"Young lady, I hope you know the advocate you have in Robert Hanover."* I chuckled and told him I hoped Robert hadn't been too hard on him, and he insisted that he had not, and once again thanked me for my patronage.

I made one more call to Denise and arranged for another nighttime pickup, but this time I booked a hotel for us at the Spokane Airport Ramada so we wouldn't have to spend two and a half hours on elk patrol in the dark. I made sure I arrived early at Tampa airport for my flight, checked in, and nervously waited for our announcement to board. Everyone at the gate was on edge, apparently with stories like mine. Our plane departed as scheduled and we made it to Minneapolis in time for our connecting flight. But as we waited for our plane to appear at the new gate, we were told we would be delayed indefinitely until our captain arrived from Detroit. And by the way, his plane was still in Detroit. My confidence wavered as we waited for our captain for nine uncomfortable airport hours, but at 10:20pm, they started boarding passengers.

We landed in Spokane a little before midnight (all twelve of us on that empty flight), and I walked over to the Ramada where Denise was already checked in, happily watching an HBO movie on her king-sized bed.

Looking back, I see how incredibly lucky I was to get on that afternoon flight. Airlines were canceling flights across the board, with existing planes less than partially full. I truly was one of the fortunate ones and just didn't know it.

We awoke early and headed straight to Rainbow Ranch in Sandpoint, about an hour-and-a-half drive. I called for an update on the way and was told that she was very sluggish and still wasn't taking any food or water. They gave me instructions to come to the back door and someone would meet me outside to gown, mask, and glove me before entering the building. I was to be the one exception to their newly enforced quarantine policy for their residents and visiting families. Pleased with that decision and clueless to the extent of precautions about to be adopted by every healthcare and assisted living facility throughout the nation, we drove on, with me anxiously anticipating seeing my mother.

As we pulled up to the back door of the building, Denise reassured me that she had her book and plenty of snacks, and that I should take as much time as I needed. She'd be right here in the parking lot waiting for me when I was ready to leave. So I clambered out of her car and shuffled my way through the snowy slush to the back door.

Something changes in you when you've worked through challenging circumstances to achieve a monumental thing and you get a glimpse of the finish line. You want it to happen NOW.

The nurse who met me at the breakroom door had been briefed on what I'd just gone through in the last 48 hours and probably had a good idea as to my current state of mind from the expression on my face. Looking back, I think we were both operating on high alert and mirrored each other's combined tension.

Neither of us had any interest in making small talk, and we wasted zero time on it. Everything I needed was stacked in a neat pile on a table just inside the door, and she instructed me to step back outside and "gown up." I couldn't remove my coat and mittens fast enough to pull my gown over my head. I twisted my hair up into the paper bonnet she handed out to me and I snapped on my gloves. *"Open,"* she instructed and shoved a thermometer under my tongue as I stood out in the cold, shivering. Twenty of the slowest seconds later, I was through the door and we were moving.

My pulse was beating through my temples, and I was sweating through my shirt under my gown as we made our way down the corridor. The nurse briefed me as we walked. She told me that my mother was in an isolation room in anticipation of my visit. They were being extra cautious, she said, because I'd come from Florida, where there was an alarming number of Coronavirus cases, and also because I'd just flown on a plane. The gravity of her words startled me. I still hadn't grasped the enormity of this pandemic or how it was about to affect our nation, or the world.

As we approached her door, she told me to take my time and to push the red button when I was ready to leave. She didn't mention how much my mother had deteriorated in the six days since her stroke or prepare me for how she now looked.

Her room was dark, and it smelled sour. She was lying on her side with Ugly Dolly under her right arm, staring blankly into its face. She didn't alter her gaze as I entered the room and knelt at the side of her bed. I wasn't sure she even knew I was there. I lowered my face to the doll's so my eyes were in line with my mother's, but she never changed her focus. Her mouth trembled, as if she was trying to speak, and her breathing was short and raspy. I touched her shoulder, hair, and took hold of her good hand and squeezed. It was cold.

She didn't respond to any of it, so I continued to talk to her through my tears. *"I'm here, Mom. Everything's going to be okay. I'm so sorry you're not feeling well."* I really didn't know what to say. I wasn't sure she could hear me or understand me, and I felt foolish, like I was reading lines from a script.

I ran out of things to say and just sat there crying. My nose was running, and it made bubbles inside my mask as I struggled to breathe through it. I tasted the salt of it as I tried not to lick my lips. I really needed a Kleenex, but I didn't move. An hour went by, and I decided to hit the red call button. The same nurse who met me at the back door popped her head in and signaled me to come toward her, where she instructed me to remove everything I'd just put on and throw it into the trash can. We stood there a moment as I struggled to collect myself, and I could see the genuine compassion on her face.

"What time tomorrow is good?" I asked as she ushered me out into the hallway.

"Oh! You can't come back into the building after this," she responded, sounding startled.

WHAT?!

"But I thought you told me you were making an exception for me," I stammered.

"We did make an exception for you, and this was it. This was your time to say goodbye. You have to understand, if the Coronavirus enters this building, it could be catastrophic with our number of compromised residents."

I took a step back, pulling my hands away as she tried to steer me further out, and sputtered, *"Then I'm going back in."* I turned around and went back inside Mom's room and closed the door behind me.

I was bawling now, completely ungowned and ungloved, and didn't know what to do with myself. My mind raced and I thought of Denise, sitting in the parking lot waiting for me. She'd assured me that she would wait for as long as it took, but my phone was inside a garbage bag with my personal things in the break room, so I couldn't call her to tell her what had just happened.

I sat back down next to the bed and watched my mother's chest rise and fall as her lungs took in air. I repeated all the things I'd already said to her, keeping my hand on her shoulder as she silently mouthed words to Ugly Dolly. We stayed this way for another hour until her eyes finally closed and she slept. This time I resolved to leave.

Knowing Denise was waiting outside in her car and uncertain what else to do with myself in Mom's room, I guess I kind-of gave up on my newly declared vigil. I pressed the red call button, the same nurse appeared at the door, and I told her I was ready to leave. I choked back sobs as we made our way down the corridor, feeling defeated while she repeated over and over how sorry she was, and I knew she was.

Denise immediately started her car and pulled forward when she saw me exit the building. She'd obviously been keeping watch for me at the back door. She came around to the passenger side and wrapped her arms around me. I leaned into her shaking, all snotty and wet, and she just hugged me. We didn't fully comprehend the health risk we were taking by riding in a vehicle together for five hours and sleeping in the same hotel room, and now I was dripping tears and mucus onto her as I wept while she held me. The whole stay-at-home directive felt like it came straight out of a Sci-Fi movie, and neither of us (or half the nation, at this point) fully took in the magnitude of this virus's deadly potential.

We rode home in silence, and she dropped me at my snowy driveway to enter my cold house that had been empty for the past six months. I had plenty of things to occupy my mind as I got everything back in order. I re-opened the water lines, bled the air out of the pipes, and turned up the heat. I made the bed, grocery shopped, and unpacked. But by the next morning, I was antsy and couldn't accept not being able to see my mother again. So after my morning call to check in on her, *"Your mother ate 10% of her dinner and nothing for breakfast. She's lethargic but responsive to stimuli."* I climbed into my truck and drove to Sandpoint to stand outside her window. At least they couldn't stop me from doing that.

I called the nurse's station from the parking lot to tell them I was outside and asked which window was hers, and would they please open the blinds, which they did within minutes. I pressed my face to the window with my hands cupped on either side, shielding the glare so I could see in. Water dripped down my neck from the roof eaves and my feet were wet from standing in a puddle of melting ice. Her mouth was closed and her eyes were open as I stood there watching her unmoving figure for about 30 minutes. The only satisfying aspect of this tragic scene was that I could unabashedly howl without fear of anyone hearing me. By now I was totally spent. And wet. I straightened myself up, wiped my nose off on my coat sleeve, and climbed back into my truck to drive home.

That afternoon I called to ask if we could use FaceTime so I could see her up close and not have to drive there to stand outside. They passed me through to the administrator and she readily agreed. Because this was new for all of us, I think everyone was willing to try just about anything as we searched for acceptable alternatives to physical visits.

For the next three days, I was able to tell her I loved her on speaker phone and get a close-up of her open-mouthed, sleeping face. Each day, the report was the same, *"Not taking food, not taking water, sleeping."*

Early Friday morning my phone rang in with "Caller ID Unknown." I don't know why I did, but I answered, thinking I could just hang up if it was another car warranty call.

The caller identified himself as Dr. Chastain from Rainbow Ranch, and I swallowed my heart. He went on to say that they had tried to administer IV fluids to my mother last night, and after several failed attempts, they gave up. He was calling to ask how I would like them to proceed. I choked out, *"Please don't stick any needles into her! I thought I had a directive that said no feeding tubes or IVs."* He confirmed that I had that directive, but he explained that I had checked the box to allow fluids, and that included IV fluids.

He offered to change it immediately and assured me that there would be no further attempts at an IV of any sort. I asked him if it was his opinion that my mother was near the end, and he replied with a calm, *"Yes."*

I could barely get the words out as I asked if there was any way I could come back to see her just one more time. He sounded surprised as he replied, *"Of course you should come see her!"*

He was silent as I told him I hadn't been allowed back in the building since my flight from Florida, and that my only way to see her these past few days was via FaceTime. I heard him draw a breath before asking me to hold the line for a moment. He returned within minutes and said, *"By all means, please come see your mother. Staff will be waiting for you at the back door when you arrive."* I think I thanked him before hanging up. I must have. But I truly don't remember anything about the end of that call.

I raced upstairs to change out of my pajamas. I forgot to brush my teeth or turn off the coffee pot as I grabbed my keys and trudged through the snow to start my truck. How I got from my driveway in Bonners Ferry to the parking lot in Sandpoint will forever be a mystery to me. It was as though I opened my eyes and was suddenly rapping on the back door, waiting to be let in.

Same neatly folded stack on the table by the door – same nurse. Only this time I was asked to leave my boots and coat outside. I hung my coat on a fence post just outside the door since neither she nor I could find anywhere else to hang it and we set my boots up against the building under an eave to keep the snow from falling into them.

The systems in place were still new and constantly changing, so everyone improvised with what information they had. No one knew exactly the correct way to proceed so we looked to each other for guidance.

Now gowned, masked, and gloved, with booties this time, I was shuffled back to Mom's room with instructions to remove myself to her bathroom and close the door whenever staff entered the room to attend to her. They were concerned that I might contaminate one of them while they were in the room with me. They could've told me to spin around five times and quack like a duck, I was following any instruction they gave if it meant I could see her again.

The final thing the nurse said to me as she opened the door to my mother's room was, *"Now the doctor DID tell you on the phone that this will be your last visit to the building and you will not be allowed to re-enter, correct?"*

NOT CORRECT!

"No! He did NOT tell me that. He told me another exception had been made for me to return because he couldn't predict how long she had left, but he said nothing about this being my final visit!"

She stood unmoving in the doorway, blocking me from my mother. Some monologue about the safety of the residents and something else about catastrophic consequences came from her masked face, but all I could do was track the rise and fall of her eyebrows, this woman who held the power over whether or not I walked through that door.

I hated everyone in that moment – the facility, this nurse, even some stupid flu that was causing all this trouble. A tear began its trail over my cheekbone, and I wiped it away in frustration before it dissolved into my mask. With clenched teeth she couldn't see, I calmly told her I understood and thanked her for her help, and she moved aside to let me pass.

I stepped into my mother's room and stopped. A horrifying mix of panic, despair, and revulsion tore through me as my eyes flitted around the room, taking in the monitors and the stacks of gauze on the bedside table. I wanted to focus on anything but her. My knee-jerk reaction to flee would've won if I hadn't just been told I wouldn't be allowed to come back.

Four days of minimal nutrition and dehydration had had a colossal effect on her, complete with gaping mouth and sunken eyes. Her head was thrown back at a grotesque angle and just barely on her pillow as she labored for shallow gasps of air. A disturbing odor that I will never forget permeated the room like a dense fog.

The door clicked shut and I was alone with her. And completely unnerved. Should I touch her? Would it hurt her if I did? Would she open her eyes and snatch my arm like they did in the movies? How do I describe the feeling of needing to flee at the exact same time as needing to stay?

"Stop it. Shake it off and help her." I pulled a chair over to her bed and forced myself to touch her. Placing my hand on her arm, her leg, then her feet, I checked everything while I told her I was there. Her feet were so cold! I found some socks for her in her drawer. Her mouth was dry and her lips were cracked. I dripped a few drops of water onto her tongue with a soaked paper towel. She began choking, unseeing eyes flying wide open as her head came off the pillow. Oh my God! I pushed the button that lifted her bed and tried to adjust her head while telling her how sorry I was when a nurse tapped on the door and peeked in.

She saw what was happening and ran in without her gown, gloves, or mask and lifted my mother into a sitting position on the bed to clear her airway. *"She can't have any water!"* she scolded, *"Anything that goes into your mother's mouth will choke her now that she's lost her ability to swallow!"* I was shaking. I don't think I responded – we just stood there looking at each other. She shook her head and began straightening the bed and organizing the bedside table.

I was in over my head. That was clear. I could've killed my mother with a few well-meaning drops of water. To that nurse I was a liability, left alone in that room with nothing but good intentions.

"Would you like me to show you how to keep your mother's mouth moist?" she asked.

"Yes, please."

She showed me how to swipe Biotine mouth hydration in

and around Mom's mouth with a sponge on a stick. Each time the sponge went into Mom's mouth she bit down on it and we had to wait a minute for her to release it before continuing.

I'd just been given my first job. And that's when I decided I wasn't leaving. Who was going to swab her mouth if I left? Who was going to sit with her?

We passed the longest day on earth together in that room, her gasping for air and me holding her hand and swabbing her mouth. There was nothing else for me to do, so I swabbed. I wanted to scream over the sounds that came from her exhausted lungs as I took breaths with her, willing the next one to be easier.

I don't think I've ever felt more lost or alone.

The sun had dropped behind the maintenance building on the other side of the parking lot, casting a shadow across the steadily darkening room. I tried the switch to her overhead lights and a harsh bluish glare invaded the room. She grimaced, so I slammed the switch down and sent us back into the dark. I sat there with her and cried. *"What can I do for you, Mom? I need you to feel better. Tell me what to do."* I'd never run a full marathon before, but that day I would've sworn I had. I'd only sat by her bedside all day, but for each breath she labored, I labored, too.

It was after 7pm when Sharon the night nurse let herself in. She stopped short when she saw me sitting in the dark.

"Who are you? I didn't know anyone was allowed in this room. I don't think you can be in here."

I told her about receiving Dr. Chastain's approval that morning and how I'd been told later that I wouldn't be allowed to come back if I left, so I'd decided to stay. I hadn't even worked out the details in my own mind yet, but I held her startled gaze as I waited to see whether I was going to have to do battle with this new nurse.

"They said that? That's terrible! I'm going to have to make

a call to confirm you can stay, though." She was back in 15 minutes. *"We had to call the Chief Administrator. You can stay."* That was the beginning of the best night-nurse-experience I will ever hope to have. She began to assess Mom and asked, *"How long has she been laboring like this?"* I told her she was like this when I arrived that morning and she hadn't changed.

"There's absolutely no need for this," she muttered.

Sharon explained that my mother had very little time left, and why not make her more comfortable? My eyes were saucers as she explained what a combination of Morphine and Ativan every four hours could do to alleviate pain and breathing anxiety in a patient during end stage, and all I remember was croaking another, *"Yes, please,"* as she left the room to go get it.

How could I have spent an entire day suffering with every strained breath she took, thinking this was just how it was? I shudder to imagine what it must've been like for her. It will be something that I'll always regret, not thinking to ask if this was normal, or whether we could make it any easier for her. I'd simply given in to the hopelessness that occupied the room with us.

I may have been a full day of agony late for that education, but I was officially on board, and I'd just been assigned my second job – timekeeper for Mom's pain relief every four hours. So I set my watch while I waited for Sharon's return.

Things can move excruciatingly slow when you're told that help is coming. It was no different with Sharon. She'd left me alone in the room again with my mother, still struggling for breath and fidgeting under the covers, but this time we were armed with a plan to fix this. So what was taking so long?!

Finally, there was a tap at the door and in popped Sharon to gown up, put on a mask, and snap on her gloves. She also had an oral syringe of morphine and the promise of Ativan in two hours. They decided to alternate the 4-hour doses so that she could have consistent and steady pain relief.

She positioned the syringe in my mother's mouth in a way that kept her from choking and pressed the plunger. I may have counted to ten. The difference in Mom's breathing was amazing and almost immediate, and we both inhaled a smooth breath with her, grinning at each other. I hiccupped my thanks to her and let every one of my tears saturate my mask.

And I re-set my watch for every two hours.

Before leaving, Sharon asked if there was anything I needed, and I told her no, that I was fine. Then she asked if I'd had any water and I admitted, *"No."* Had I eaten? *"No."* She moved toward the door and told me she'd be right back. Then she disrobed, de-masked, ungloved, threw everything into the can, and left. Twenty minutes later, there was a tap on the door and Sharon leaned in with a tray of the best split pea soup and crackers I've ever tasted, a gorgeous apple, and an ice cold bottle of water. No doubt she could hear my stomach growling as she slid the tray into the room.

I stopped her before she disappeared behind the door and asked if she would write down a phone number. I needed her to call Sam, the only number I could remember, to tell him where I was and ask him to call Denise. She'd know who else to call.

"My cell phone's in the pocket of my coat with my keys. I had to leave everything outside this morning, so we hung my coat on the fence post out by the staff entrance." I explained. She shook her head, incredulous, *"I saw that coat when I got here tonight – it's covered in snow and your boots are full of water. I wondered why they were out there."* Then she promised me she'd be right back and closed the door.

Twenty more minutes passed and Sharon was at the door. She reached in, holding a clear sealed bag containing my disinfected cell phone, a blanket, a sheet, and a pillow. *"No one should have to go through this,"* she tisked. *"Keep the phone put away, but use it to contact your people and let them know where you are."* Are you waiting for me to tell you that I stood there sobbing? I certainly did.

The angst-ridden day I'd just spent alone with my mother and my imagination had filled my head with visions of my stolen truck, sure credit card theft, and a subsequent home invasion. Pile on my inability to ease my mother's unrelenting discomfort, and I was one wrecked individual. So with the miraculous introduction of Morphine, some food, my phone, and nurse Sharon's kindness, my flood gates opened wide.

Things were looking up (as much as things do). My soup bowl was empty, and my phone calls were made, so I was free to focus on my second job of managing Ativan and Morphine schedules. It was time for her first Ativan dose and Sharon appeared before I needed to press the red call button. My heart was full. I settled in for an endlessly long night in an automatic reclining chair that didn't in fact recline, listening for any reason to press the red call button and saying hello to Sharon every two hours.

The room was still dark when I opened my eyes the next morning. I blinked them into focus and searched for my mother. She was still in the same position, on her side and peacefully breathing. Every muscle ached along my back, and my eyes burned from the puffs of air that escaped the top of my mask with each exhaled breath. I'd made the mistake of not removing my gloves since I'd arrived the morning before, and instead just washed my gloved hands to keep from using up the nurses' now-coveted supply. I finally took them off and my hands were wet and smelled like feet. I must have washed them five times to rid them of the foulness.

Kitchen staff were coming and going outside her courtyard window now, and as our room began to fill with light, I watched them unload boxes from a delivery truck. There was a shuffling outside the door and someone in a mask and gown stuck his head in, motioning for me to step toward the door and take the Styrofoam container and insulated coffee pot from him. He chirped, *"Good morning! We heard you were in here!"* and backed away. Someone had drawn a smiley face on top of the container with a Sharpie pen and wrote, *"Fay's daughter."* I opened the lid to a beautiful pile of cheesy scrambled eggs, bacon, and toast. My coffee was hot, and I'd never enjoyed powdered coffee creamer more in my life.

Sharon was gone. I'd slept through her last Morphine delivery and didn't get to say goodbye. I looked at my watch and jerked upright with the realization that we were half an hour behind on Mom's Ativan. I reached for the red call button and stopped. Did I really want a rocky start with the new nurse? I already knew what my first red-call-button-request-for-drugs at the beginning of her shift would prompt her to think. *"This is going to be one of 'those daughters' kinds of shifts today."* So I pressed it anyway.

She rapped on the door and snapped, *"Can I help you with something?"* I took one deep breath and said, *"Good morning. I'm Fay's daughter."* I explained that my only job in this room was to manage my mother's pain care, and that we were 30 minutes past due, so I thought I would send out the call. She asked if my mother was showing signs of distress, since the order was for "every four hours as needed."

Prepared now, I explained that my opinion would remain the same – that it *was* needed, and that I would continue to watch the clock every two hours in order to help her out with the split doses. Her eyes never left mine as she explained that she'd been busy with the beginning demands of her shift and that I'd see her again in two hours after this dose, and I did. A little while later, she brought me a toothbrush, toothpaste, deodorant, and a dry shampoo cap. I could tell we were going to be friends.

Later that morning I received a text from Sam, asking how

things were. I responded that today was much better, and that she was so much more peaceful. His return text read, *"Tell her it's okay for her to go."* I read it again. I'd been telling her that I was there, that everything was going to be okay, and that I wasn't going to leave. But tell her to actually *go*? How did he expect me to say something like that? And out loud! *"Hey Mom, it's okay, just, you know... go."* I felt like a monumental fraud saying it. Where do we "go," anyway?

My religious beliefs are pretty minimal, I'll admit. I mentioned earlier that I was raised in the church. But sometime later, as an adult, I lost my faith and sided with science, choosing to live a good, moral life, but not a faith-based one. So I tucked the phone back into its hiding place and slid the chair to the other side of her bed where she was facing. I eased myself down, never taking my eyes off her fluttering lashes, and contemplated what to do next. Wrapping my hands around hers, I started to talk. I pushed past my discomfort and ignored the hollow sound of my voice as I told her how comfortable she was in her soft bed with clean sheets and a cool pillow; that she could just sink into it and float away.

I talked about all the people waiting to see her and described each one. *"Okay, I can do it like this,"* I thought. I reminded her how much fun we had when she came out to Idaho for the first time and I surprised her by bringing Aunt Jack out from Portland. I retold the story of how Dad built her a set of Adirondack chairs for her birthday and surprised her with them on the back porch. And how her sister, Aunt Sis, had brought her to New York City where she met him in the first place, so young, from Kansas. I recalled smelt fishing with Aunt Darlene in Oregon, and our summer trip to see Aunt Lois and her rabbits in Michigan. Even her favorite dog, Gigi, was bouncing up and down to see her. When I ran out of stories I started over again, helping her picture their excited faces, and how peaceful it must feel to just relax and float to them.

I finally turned on the TV and watched the Covid-19 coverage that was broadcasting throughout the day on CNN. A PBS special on the March of Dimes and their fight against Polio was on when a tap at the door produced another Styrofoam box donning a happy face, presented by the same chipper person who delivered breakfast. This time it was a ham sandwich, pear, and a bag of chips. I ate my lunch on the end of my mother's bed and smiled just knowing there were people keeping watch over me close by in the kitchen.

With freshly brushed teeth and a new set of gloves, I wiped down the bed frame and my chair with the sanitizing wipes a nurse left earlier. None of our attempts at disinfecting the room seemed to eradicate the stale smell that surrounded me like a cloak. Her stack of mouth sponges was dwindling and I made a note to ask for more the next time a nurse came in. There was nothing left to do while I waited for her Morphine and Ativan arrivals, so I settled myself next to her and started reciting the story of her life from the beginning.

Evening eased in as the sun resumed its path behind the maintenance building, and I finished her story in the dark. I turned the TV back on and muted the volume. The eerie flicker it cast across my mother's face was unsettling, but I couldn't risk upsetting her again with the harsh overhead lights.

Dinner came with another gentle rap on the door and another Styrofoam box, this time with a cup of pudding. The artist in the kitchen was getting more elaborate, and I chuckled at the smiling flower surrounded by bumblebees and puffy clouds. I imagined their grin had to be as big while creating as mine was while receiving.

I had just finished my turkey, gravy, and stuffing when I noticed a change in Mom's breathing. The nurse had been in with her Ativan just before my box arrived, so it didn't make sense that she'd be anything but peaceful. I went to the side of her bed and whispered, *"What's wrong, Mom?"*

Something was different. I reached for the red button on the wall and pushed it. If there was a higher dose of something for her, I was asking for it. We'd been doing so well all day, and I wasn't going to chance a repeat of yesterday's misery.

The red light flashed above her head while we waited together. *"Hang in there, Mom. Someone's coming to make things easier for you."* I began reminiscing about our holidays together and chose Halloween, for some reason. I hadn't gotten past our pumpkin carving chaos on the kitchen table when I noticed she'd become completely still. I fell silent and stared at her chest. It wasn't moving. I didn't realize I'd been holding my breath along with her and finally exhaled a soft, *"It's okay Mom. You can go now."*

I watched her for another minute and leaned closer, searching her face for any sign of movement when she suddenly drew in a huge gulp of air. Her eyes flew open, body stiffened, and back arched so drastically that she nearly lifted off the bed. I sprang backward, tipping my chair over, and lunged toward the door to get help.

I yanked the door open to an empty hallway. It was break time, dinner time, who knew – but there was no one around. As I contemplated breaking the rules and rushing out into the common area for help, I glanced back over my shoulder at her and saw that she'd relaxed back onto the bed and was completely still again.

Somehow I knew this was the beginning of her leaving and I let the door shut with a click. I turned to look at her, unwilling to let go of the handle. *"Move!"* I screamed inside my head as I took the steadying breath I needed to return to the side of her bed. *"What should I do, Mom? How can I make this better for you?"*

I suddenly knew beyond anything else in my life that I needed to help her go. The red call light continued to flash, and this time I reached over and turned it off. The last thing I wanted now was a nurse bursting through the door and robbing me of these last moments with her.

She stayed completely still for the longest time. I held my breath again, bracing myself for that backwards jerk and horrific gasp for air, and she did. This time I didn't jump. I just kept talking. I told her to relax her shoulders and take a nice deep breath. That the bed was so soft and comfortable for her. I told her she was the best mother, and that I could never have chosen a better one. That the person I had become was all because of her. I asked her to please keep her eye on me from up there. I told her I'd continue to talk to her from down here, and if she could, to send me a message that she could hear me.

I surprised myself because I realized I meant it. I sat with her, crying over my loss and her relief, until I was sure she wasn't going to gasp one last time. I touched her arm, and it was cool, but her face was still warm. Her eyes wouldn't stay closed and her mouth was open. I smoothed her quilt as I busily wiped my tears from its surface and finally pressed the red call button.

It took a while for the tap on the door, and this time I didn't care. I had no tears left and I was just peacefully sitting with her. The nurse poked her head in, and I watched her glance between me and my mother. She said she'd be right back and went to get another caregiver. They came in and I removed myself to the bathroom. I could hear them adjusting the bed, straightening things, and cooing to Mom as they worked. It wasn't long before they tapped on the bathroom door to say I could come out, and I entered the room to find my mother laying perfectly in her bed. Her hands were crossed, eyes closed (how did they manage that?), and her hair was combed.

"Take as much time with her as you need," they said in unison as they moved to the door. I wasn't even sure what that meant – minutes? hours? Everything was different now,

foreign, and so quiet. Even the staff noises in the hallway outside the door seemed to be gone, maybe out of respect for my mother, I wasn't sure. She was right there in front of me, but she wasn't, and I couldn't figure out how I felt. I'd just spent two full days in agony with her, wishing for it to be over. And now that it was, the only thing I knew was that I didn't want to leave her. Instead, I kissed her forehead, thanked her for being my mother, and for the last time, I pressed the red call button.

They found my coat and keys, but no one knew where my boots were. It was Saturday night, and no one had the key to the administrator's office where someone had last seen them. I didn't want to speak with anyone yet, so I took out my phone and sent some texts while they searched for my boots. I sat with her for another 15 or 20 minutes until they finally found them.

We made awkward company as we shuffled down the hall together, this nurse I'd never met. She, trying to gauge my emotions and say just the right things, and me, in a fog and not hearing anything she said. I removed my gown, mask, gloves, and booties outside the back entrance door as instructed, placed them in the bag she held out for me, and walked the parcel to the dumpster outside. I think she said something about how sorry she was and how they'd all loved Fay, and I think I said thank you or some other thankful thing.

I climbed into my ice-covered truck and started it in the dark, turning up the heat. My phone began to ping and I read my texts while I waited for the windshield to defrost. From Robert – (we'd remained close friends since we ended things a few years earlier) *"Looks like it's snowing there on my weather app. Please don't drive home alone."* From Denise – *"Please let me come get you. It's no trouble."* From John – (my new boyfriend in Florida) *"Please ride home with Denise."*

From Sam – *"I'm coming to get you. Let me know when you're ready."*

So I backed the truck out of the parking lot and drove home in the dark.

POSTSCRIPT.

It's been months since my mother left. I'd be lying if I said I was a basket case this whole time. After that initial night, I've only had some random sobbing outbursts, mostly over within a few minutes. Should I be more distraught than I am? How long should the tears last? Am I supposed to announce it on Facebook? That conflict between what is true and what is expected is alive and well within me.

I didn't write an obituary for our local paper. Why, when there's no one in my town who was close to her except the people in this story, and they were all "with me" when she died.

I still haven't told many people she died, even though so many were aware that she was my main focus and priority for eight years. When they ask how she's doing, I tell them then. I'm usually met with a look of surprise, sometimes hurt, and other times even guilt that they'd missed that significant event in my life. But whichever I see, it's always quickly replaced by sincere sympathy.

I contacted the cousins privately, most through text. Each responded with love for my mother and sadness over my loss; these people I haven't seen in over 30 years, and some I've never met. They informed their respective mothers, her two remaining sisters. One also has dementia and likely won't comprehend.

Mom's body was cremated, and I chose the basic cardboard box option for her instead of a lovely urn, why again? She's no longer here, in my eyes, and the thought of her packed inside some ornate vase on my mantel unnerves me. I'll scatter her ashes together with Dad's (we'd managed to lose him and find him again several times during my mother's moves), but I haven't yet decided where. Right now she's on a shelf in the back of a closet with him. I'm not ready to see either of them, truthfully.

Weird things happened for weeks after her death that I didn't share with anyone. I sometimes caught the movement of a figure behind me as I sat on the couch at night. Or my hair would blow a little off my shoulder while doing dishes. I'd always rolled my eyes when people reported these sorts of experiences in the past. As if they made them up because it was the popular thing to say, setting them apart from the boring survivors who felt nothing. But I understood it now.

I finally mentioned it to Robert. He knows me well enough to know I'd never believe it if it weren't actually happening to me. I wasn't outright afraid, since doors weren't slamming and lights weren't flickering, but I was unnerved, especially at night. *"You know, it might be Fay,"* he suggested. *"Why don't you tell her it's okay to continue along on her journey?"* Just the kind of thing I'm not comfortable with, but after several more incidents, I decided to try.

It didn't take long for me to see her again, and I was prepared. I took a big breath, swallowed, and began speaking the words out loud that I'd been practicing in my head. *"Hi MeeMaw. Thank you for checking on me. I miss you, but I'm going to be fine. You should continue on now. Everyone's waiting for you."* I remember speaking to her twice.

Those were the times I burst out crying, sobbing for my mother. Talking to an apparition was unsettling enough, but intentionally scripting directives for her to move along made her absence that much more definitive.

I can't say I noticed an immediate change, but one night I realized I hadn't seen her in a while, and I knew then that she really was gone. As relieved as I was not to be jarred alert on quiet evenings anymore by a reflection behind me in the window, her departure left me feeling hollow.

I was driving home from the gym this morning and spotted an elderly woman scooting up Mom's hill at a good clip with a bag in each hand, hunkered over the weight of it. I was instantly thrust back in time, and I worried for her and her family. Did they know she was out here on this stretch of road alone? Where was she going? Did *she* even know where she was going? Was she loved? By the time I reached a point where I could turn my truck around and head back down the hill, she was gone. Did some good Samaritan pick her up? Or did she turn onto a different street? I was left with an emptiness and feeling of forlorn after seeing her, recognizing the extent of the journey she and her family might be about to take, or were already on.

So I turned back around and drove home.

$\mathcal{A}$FTERWORD.

TALKING WITH FAY

Two of my girlfriends call me on a pretty regular basis these days to vent about their moms. Both mothers have dementia, one with Lewy Body and the other is undiagnosed. The uncanny thing is that almost every situation they find themselves in mirrors some interaction I've had with my own mother. Their calls always begin with our usual catching-up but invariably move on to some difficult scenario they've recently found themselves in with their moms, followed with, *"I can't believe I responded that way to her! Everything went downhill from there. Did this ever happen to you?"*

Midway through their detailed recounting of their latest atrocity, I'll catch myself nodding my head while conjuring a memory of being in my own mother's shooting range. I always let them finish, give them a moment to recover from their shock and indignation, and then offer my opinion.

The curious thing I've noticed is oftentimes we'll end up doing this dance where I share with them a similar scenario of how it went wrong with my mother, suggest a better response for them to use next time, and then spend the rest of the call gently arguing with them why their chosen tactic caused the unfortunate outcome it did and why it shouldn't be repeated, right, wrong, or otherwise. Even the most innocent, *"Mom! You've asked me that question ten times today!"* is a reaction nearly impossible for the novice to stifle. So when I hear the more offensive accusations of random theft and premeditated cruelty, I settle in for what I know is going to be an even lengthier conversation.

Neither of my friends wants to accept that it's okay to *"repeatedly take the abuse"* (their words). Their need to expose the injustice meted out to them and insist their mothers listen to reason is overpowering, and they cling to their strongly justified approach. Just like I once did.

The fact is no one likes to be accused of a crime they didn't commit. There's nothing more dissatisfying than sitting through a character assault and choosing not to defend yourself. And even more objectionable is being the recipient of that judgment from the person you love.

The more we compared stories and even our initial reactions, the more it began to feel like Groundhog Day. It reinforced in me again the need for a truthful, no-nonsense accounting of what can (and likely will) happen as you proceed down your loved one's own path into dementia.

So I began creating a list of conversations I remembered having with my mother, complete with my mistakes, my successes, and their outcomes. Maybe you'll read even one that sticks with you when you need it most.

"How old are you now?"

- I'm 50, Mom. Can you believe your youngest child is that old?

"You can't be that old! I'm only 40!"

Truth: "No Mom, you're 83. You were born in 1932."

Better: "Huh! Who would've thought? You look great for 40!"

What really happened: Reminding her she was 83 sent her into immediate distress. She demanded to see a mirror. When presented with one, she stared into it while repeatedly touching her face and whispering, *"Oh. Oh. Oh."* She pummeled me with questions about my father and where he was and then grieved his death each time I answered truthfully (another regret) that he'd died several years prior. When I chose the "better" response the next time she asked, she happily carried on like any 40-year-old would and we ate sandwiches together.

"Why haven't you given me any grandkids?"
  - I guess I just never wanted a baby, Mom.
  "Well, that was selfish. Now I'll have to have one for you."
  <u>Truth</u>: "You've always criticized me for not having children! And that's ridiculous to say you'll have to have one for me when you know it's impossible."
  <u>Better</u>: "Well, maybe I can babysit for you when you do. That would be nice."
  <u>What really happened</u>: She got very quiet when I responded with the truth and lunch was ruined. Once I tried the "better" response, we spent the rest of our conversation happily discussing baby names, boy/girl preferences, and reminiscing over my adoption stories.

"Where's my car? I know you have it somewhere!"
  <u>Truth</u>: "It's at an auto shop back in Georgia being listed for sale because you don't drive safely anymore."
  <u>Better</u>: "It's in the shop. You must've hit something and it needs an alignment."
  <u>What really happened</u>: Telling her she could no longer drive was a huge mistake. Adding the fact that I was selling her car was even worse. She was furious with me and fixated on it for weeks, calling me a liar, and schemer, and jailer. I'd read somewhere about "putting the car in the shop," and was sure she'd never believe my completely altered story the next time she hurled her accusation that I'd stolen her car and left her stranded, but she did! Straight-faced I tried it, and like magic she immediately calmed down, quipping, *"Well, I know I didn't hit anything, but let them look it over if they want to."*

"Look at you! Again on the cover of this magazine!"

Truth: "That's Queen Latifah, Mom."

What really happened: I can't count how many magazine covers my face graced during the time my mom was at The Community Resting Place (for some reason, I was only famous while she lived there and was hoarding them in her drawers). It was easy enough to go along with her insistence that I was Julia Roberts, Kate Hudson, or any number of beauties, so why not? She'd ask me questions about my outfits, and I'd launch into lengthy descriptions of my photo shoots.

"I know you came into my house last night and stole my things. All of my quilts are missing!"

Truth: "You know I didn't come into your house! How can you accuse me of stealing from you after everything I've done for you?!"

Better: "Let's look for your quilts together. I'm sure we can find them."

What really happened: She met me at the door most mornings calling me a thief. It was a terrible way to start our visits (and my mornings). I learned the "better" tactic from one of my AA meetings, and it worked the first time I tried it. We searched together, found her quilts in any number of places, and then laid them out on the bed together while she pointed out unusual patterns and pretty colors, her venomous accusations instantly forgotten. We typically went hunting for items "I stole from her last night" once or twice a week. I got good at finding them inside the oven, under beds, and even stuffed into the chest freezer.

***Note: It took LOTS of practice to get over my hurt feelings from her character assaults. I had to continually remind myself that the peaceful outcome far outweighed my need for vindication, because I certainly wasn't going to get an apology. Did I want to pout after finding her stolen quilts, sniping, *"Oh! I* *thought you said I'd stolen them! See?? How does that make you feel now, Mom?"* Yes, more than anything, I did.

"How could you take me from my home and put me here?! I want to go home! Now!"

Truth: "You can't live on your own anymore, Mom. You're a danger to yourself. This is your home now."

Better: "Show me the pretty photos of your garden again. I've always loved how you cared for it." And later still, "Dale is coming to get you. He's putting in for vacation time and then he'll come."

What really happened: I never did tell her this truth. I didn't have the guts or the heart for it, and I lied to her from the beginning. Most times, diversion worked best, until it didn't. I finally invented the story of my brother Dale coming out to get her after a particularly relentless day of questioning and the tale just seemed to come together naturally. Once she knew Dale was coming, she didn't care so much about "why" she was there, and I could skip right past that; it was enough that he was coming to get her. No matter how many times she assaulted me with her demands to go home, reminding her that Dale was coming would instantly calm her.

"When is Dale coming to get me and bring me home?" (for the hundredth time)

Truth: "Dale was a raging alcoholic, and he passed away last year. He never visited you unless he needed something from you, anyway, Mom, so why do you think he'd come all this way for you now?

Better: "He's putting in for vacation time and planning his trip out here as we speak."

What really happened: Telling my mother that alcoholism took her son's life would've crushed her, so I never told her. He remained her savior for the rest of her life. I could put any spin on Dale's trip out west, from his vacation time being delayed, to truck problems, to a simple, *"Any day now."* Any excuse was fine as long as I finished it with an unblinking, *"He's on his way."*

The key with my mother was to figure out what made her happy. What reassured her. In this case, knowing that her son was coming to save her was all she needed.

A friend of a friend stopped me the other day with, *"Hey, I heard you're writing a book about your mother. I just lost my mom this summer. She had dementia, too."* I told him how sorry I was, and he shared with me his regret that he couldn't be with her when she died because she refused to see him. I was struck by his statement and asked why she wouldn't see him. His response? *"The last year of her life we had to put her in a memory care facility. She begged me to come take her home. I finally told her that she was sick and needed to stay there until they could make her better. She never spoke to me again after that."* It was too late to suggest a different way for him to respond to her, and I don't know whose heart mine broke for more, his or hers.

"What did you do with all of my things? I can't find my sewing machine/red blouse/juice glasses..."

Truth: "We couldn't fit everything in the moving van, so we had to pitch a lot of your things in the dumpster."

Better: "Tomorrow I'll help you look for your things. Want to help me make lunch? I'm in the mood for grilled cheese sandwiches!"

What really happened: That sewing machine? No amount of diversion helped it go away, and I tried everything. Out of desperation, I called the person I gave it to in Georgia and explained my situation. She was wonderful. She boxed it up, sewing cabinet and all, and seven days later Mom's sewing machine miraculously appeared in her basement. My mother was perplexed when we spotted it in the corner and swore it wasn't there when she checked earlier, but she was pleased as punch to see it. Interestingly, she never mentioned it again after that, never touched it again, and I was out $225 in freight shipping fees.

"My neighbors are spying on me and stealing my mail from my mailbox. I'm going to call the police!"

Truth: "How can you say that about your nice neighbors!? They would never steal from you! They keep an eye on you for me when I can't be here!"

Better: "I'll go talk with them about being so nosey. Let's close your curtains tonight."

What really happened: I tried the truth first, like most rookies. I couldn't stand to hear her say those things about such caring people who constantly looked out for her and showed her incredible kindness. The truth simply enraged her. Hearing that people were "keeping an eye on her" only heightened her anxiety. She accused me of plotting against her with these strangers and became fixated on the elderly couple across the street. They finally called me one day to ask that I keep my mother off their property, stating she'd been sneaking over every morning (yes, in full daylight and easily viewed from their kitchen window) and emptying their mailbox.

"I hate it here! They're mean to me. They starve us! And one of them is stealing from me."

Truth: "Here we go again, Mom. Everyone is always stealing from you. I'm sick of hearing about it. And no one is being mean to you. They're all so nice! They serve three meals a day, and you just finished lunch."

Better: "Oooh! I smell fresh coffee! Let's walk over to the coffee cart and get the first cup before anyone else. Maybe we can find you a snack to go along with it."

<u>What really happened</u>: My mother could be wiping her mouth and pushing back her plate while insisting she hadn't eaten anything all day. Same with her bottomless cup of coffee. There were days she'd have her nearly empty cup perched next to her, insisting they were refusing to serve her coffee. If I pointed out her cup, she'd swear someone had just put that next to her to prove her wrong. Nothing was right in her mind on those days and the only thing that worked was distraction. When I practiced, I could sense it early enough to think of something nice to offer her instead.

And of course, saving the best for last. *"How did I raise you to be such a despicable, greedy daughter? I never thought I'd see the day my own daughter would steal/lie/cheat/ scheme against me."*

<u>Truth</u>: (The outrage! Insert any number of wounded retorts here, because I had plenty.)

<u>Better</u>: There were times (like these) when diversion simply didn't work during a full and direct frontal assault. And "Look! A bear!" certainly didn't make sense. But a clean, "I'm so sorry, Mom. I want to do better, and I will try harder," blew the wind right out of her sails almost every time, and we had peace again.

<u>What really happened</u>: It took dozens of do-overs before I finally acquiesced to the simple apology. My pride kept me from accepting it as an option because I couldn't accept the thought of asking for forgiveness for a crime I hadn't committed. And in truth, I dreaded her response. I was terrified she would take it and run with it, snapping, *"That's right! You ARE a terrible daughter! And you call that trying?! You're such a disappointment."*

It took someone in my AA meeting to offer, *"So what if she says that? Maybe it's exactly what she needs to express right now. Help her get it off her chest. Have you considered how*

*powerless she must be feeling? In her mind, you've taken
everything from her. Why not grant her this tongue-lashing
opportunity and see what she does with it? Besides, she won't
remember it tomorrow."*

They were right, and my worst fear never came true. Not
once did she respond with anything other than a self-satisfied
expression and a conversational clean slate. She would
amazingly carry on with any unrelated topic of the day, and
we'd proceed as though her outburst never happened. The
hardest part was the apology and letting go of the sting of the
accusation – both things within my control. And I was given
plenty of opportunities to get it right.

When I reflect on all my conversations with Fay, I know
one thing. She truly and unequivocally believed whatever she
said was true. Every bit of it. Dementia did that to her. It
altered her reality in ways that left her grappling for logical
explanations (logical to her, anyway) to make sense of it, and
she managed to do it. No amount of reasoning from me or
anyone else could convince her otherwise.

This has become the root of my phone conversations with
my two girlfriends. They've begun to see an ugly side of their
mothers they never thought existed. They insist on explaining
reality to them, trying endlessly to help their moms see
reason. Why? Because the ugly side is ugly. It makes them
uncomfortable, and they want it to stop.

They don't like this new person inside their mother's body,
and who can blame them? Random glimpses of the "old
version" give them just enough proof that she's still in there
to keep them from simply accepting this imposter and getting
on with the task of caring for her needs. Their suspicion that
their moms know full well what they're doing and are
behaving this way on purpose is so compelling that they
continue to turn to it as a possibility. I remember it well.

I wondered out loud on the phone one day how my friend's

visits might go if she began by presenting a small gift to her mother when she arrived. Just a little something to derail her mother's rage-train. For my mom, the prize was fruit, so I got in the habit of meeting her at the door with an extended palm holding a massive apple or gorgeous orange. She would exclaim over its beauty, forget what she was about to shout at me, and we would often have an in-depth conversation about that piece of fruit for the duration of our visit. Bullet dodged.

If I had one wish, I think it would be that I could go back to the beginning with my mother. I wish I would've recognized that her accusations and endless rounds of questioning were her way of saying, *"I'm scared. Things aren't making sense to me. I feel powerless."* Maybe then I would've spent less time volleying back each serve and more time figuring out what she really needed at that moment instead.

"What's wrong, Mom? What can I do for you right now to make you smile?"

"You want to go home? Okay, I'll work on it, and we'll get you home."

"Your money's missing? Let's go check the mail, but first let's grab our shoes so we can go see if the flowers opened yet in your garden on our way to the mailbox."

"Someone stole your yellow jacket? Let's go see if they dropped it in the coat closet while trying to make their escape."

I wish I'd had both the confidence in my conviction that my mother's disease and her true nature were two separate things, and the emotional capacity to recognize the difference. That the next terrible thing she said to me or her newest abhorrent behavior wouldn't send my feelings of affection for her spiraling south when really, she was just in her most confused and frightened state and merely striking out.

I wish (okay, that's more than one wish) I'd had the patience and humor to roll with her moods and quirks with more genuine kindness and empathy. I may have outwardly been caring for my mother, but I spent years inwardly seething over the injustice of suffering her abuse – a huge regret. I repeatedly forgot that, in her mind, I wasn't protecting her from all the things that felt so wrong. In fact, every decision I made in order to keep her safe felt like a betrayal to her, and her only way to regain some sense of power was to lash out at me. And every time I tried to help her "see," I became the conniving enemy.

And now that she's gone, I don't get another do-over, and I'd like just one more, maybe two.

So, shampoo, rinse, and repeat, my friend. Don't be afraid to modify your stroke until you find the one that works. And when that one stops working, search for another. Your real objective is to bring peace to your loved one during a tremendously frightening time for them.

Some visits with my mother were so trying that I reworked my storyline five or six times in one sitting. It was frustrating beyond belief, and there were plenty of times I lost my patience. On a good day, I'd remind myself to aim for that look of calm on her face that for one short moment signaled I'd gotten it right. On a bad day, I'd lose it and line drive whatever she was serving right back at her. And I got plenty of practice. There were days when she fired away at me on a 60 second loop until I found the right response or I gave up and walked out. But when I succeeded, her shoulders would relax, and she'd reward me with a smile. It was like a balm to her wounds and a small triumph for me.

Deflection, distraction, and well-crafted fibs became my saviors once I mastered them, and maybe hers, too.

*T*HINGS THAT HELPED ME.

<u>Alzheimer's Association</u>

<u>www.alz.org</u>

The Alzheimer's Association's website, www.alz.org, is an incredible source of information. To find local meetings in your area, select "Local Resources" at the top of the page and enter your zip code for local chapters. This group became my lifeline. They helped me feel more normal and provided great ideas along the way.

<u>My family and friends</u>

Remember that they love you. And they're probably as much at a loss over what to do as you are, but they *do* want to help. Take more breaths and count to ten more often than I did. Those closest to you only want to make your pain go away and are your most valuable allies. How they deliver their support may not feel like the help you need right then, so try to tell them what does. Find a way if you can. Because when this is all over (and it will be, I promise) and your loved one is gone, those closest to you will still be here (if you don't fall prey to all the craziness and push them away). And you're going to need them.

<u>Psychology Today</u> (Definition of anger-guilt splits)

<u>www.psychologytoday.com/us/blog/theory-knowledge/201305/understanding-anger-guilt-splits</u>

Anger and guilt are social emotions that are activated as a function of social exchange. Anger is activated when we perceive the social exchange to be in the other person's favor. That is, the kinds of situations that activate the emotion of anger:

- When we perceive ourselves as being treated unfairly
- When our interests are not being respected
- When we are not heard
- When we are not deferred to when we have legitimate authority
- When someone who owes us fails to repay us
- When we are not given what we believe we are entitled to, or similar such situations
- In short, when others devalue our interests relative to what we perceive we deserve, we get angry

Guilt, in contrast, is activated when we perceive ourselves to be overly self-centered and not as concerned as we ought to be with the feelings or interests of others. Guilt results in an anxious feeling that keeps us from acting selfishly, orients us toward seeking the approval of important others, and allows us to maintain an affiliative, connected stance with the other. Indeed, when people feel guilty, they often will want to make amends by giving or doing something for others...

Alzheimer's Weekly

www.alzheimersweekly.com

I loved this website! Sort of like an online magazine on dementia with interesting articles and helpful tips.

Teepa Snow's Positive Approach to Care

www.teepasnow.com

Oh my gosh, every caregiver *everywhere* should watch her videos, in my opinion. A lightbulb went off in my head when I watched her gentle, logical approach to interacting with someone with dementia.

Today's Caregiver

www.caregiver.com

This website is dedicated to caregivers in every arena, whether it's dementia, cancer, stroke, or other medical condition, they focus on the health and emotional well-being of those caring for others.

DailyCaring

www.dailycaring.com

This is where I found the tips to deal with my mom's endless accusations by typing "accusations" in the search bar. I was shocked to find that nearly every one she pummeled me with was in these examples.

A Place for Mom

www.aplaceformom.com

This is where I found the article that explained the five ways the elderly cover up the signs of their dementia.

Melissa and Doug Toys

www.melissaanddoug.com

Seriously. My mother was enamored with these colorful wooden activity boards and could sit with them for endless hours of entertainment.

<u>Ashton Drake Lifelike Baby Dolls</u>

<u>www.ashtondrake.com</u>

They now have several baby dolls to choose from, which is a nice addition since I first happened upon Dolly. As time went on, my mother fell in love with any sort of baby doll, plastic, ugly, or otherwise, but it was nice to present her with such a realistic baby that one Christmas.

$\mathcal{M}$ANY THANKS.

I'm a fortunate girl. I'm surrounded by friends who not only love me, but who immediately believed in me when I told them I was writing this book. From each of you, I received similar suggestions, conflicting advice, and polar opposite reactions to so many aspects of my story that I couldn't help but craft the most well-rounded final version I could've hoped for.

Ginny Kirsch, you get the award for the sharpest eagle eyes ever. Steve Dickinson, my toughest critic and biggest fan, I couldn't wait to open your revisions and read your feedback. Alicia Charland, you swore you never got tired of reading each draft, and I think I finally believe you! Mary Beth Watkins, your wish list kept me on my toes and forced me to re-visit areas of the book I thought I'd put to bed, and I thank you for that. Lynn Silva, hearing your "wow!" in all the right places reinforced for me that I was on the right track. Laura Richardson, you never stopped cheerleading. Delia Owens, I named Draft Four my "Delia Draft" and doubled my word count after finally understanding the difference between showing and telling that you helped me see. And Lynn Piecuch, every question you asked helped me to better construct my thoughts on paper.

To John Birrell, who out-witted my every excuse not to write by installing a 3pm daily alarm in my cell phone calendar with simply, *"WRITE."* How many opportunities did you find to celebrate my every accomplishment? I've lost count.

To my Beta Readers: Sue Kirkland, Rana Campbell, Gail Brown, Carrie Figgins, Jori Fahrenfeld, Doreen DeRoy, Willow Feller, Ruth Ann Milby – each of you jumped right in and read.

And your feedback helped shape this book.

And saving the best for last, Denise Crichton, Ginny Kirsch, Robert Hanover, Sam Testa, Roxanne Furnace, Rhonda Hamerslough, Jolle Wall, Kim Casey and Betty Edwards, you helped me fill these pages while you filled my life with love and support during a time when I needed you, whether you knew it then or not.

$\mathcal{A}$BOUT ATMOSPHERE PRESS

Atmosphere Press is an independent, full-service publisher for excellent books in all genres and for all audiences. Learn more about what we do at atmospherepress.com.

We encourage you to check out some of Atmosphere's latest releases, which are available at Amazon.com and via order from your local bookstore:

The Swing: A Muse's Memoir About Keeping the Artist Alive, by Susan Dennis

Possibilities with Parkinson's: A Fresh Look, by Dr. C

Gaining Altitude - Retirement and Beyond, by Rebecca Milliken

Out and Back: Essays on a Family in Motion, by Elizabeth Templeman

Just Be Honest, by Cindy Yates

You Crazy Vegan: Coming Out as a Vegan Intuitive, by Jessica Ang

Detour: Lose Your Way, Find Your Path, by S. Mariah Rose

To B&B or Not to B&B: Deromanticizing the Dream, by Sue Marko

Convergence: The Interconnection of Extraordinary Experiences, by Barbara Mango and Lynn Miller

ABOUT THE AUTHOR

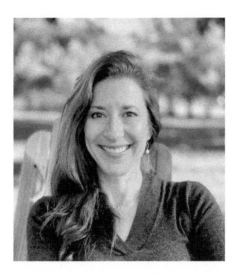

Carolyn Birrell retired to Bonners Ferry, ID, after living in Atlanta, GA, for 20 years, where she worked for the American Cancer Society National Headquarters and then as a real estate agent and new home builder. She began caring for her aging mother shortly after her move and started chronicling her journey. What began as a written collection of her mother's difficult behaviors during dementia's earliest stages quickly turned into a comprehensive book that she continued to update until the inevitable end of her mother's disease. She now balances her time between the amazing Gem State and the Florida Gulf Coast, where you can usually find her on her paddle board, plucking strings on her ukulele, or pulling weeds. For more information, visit www.carolynbirrell.com. This is her first book.

Thank you for reading my story!
I hope you'll take a few moments to review it.

This QR code will take you directly to my website,
www.carolynbirrell.com, *where you'll find links to several*
book sellers from whom you may have purchased your copy.
Just point your phone camera at it!

carolynbirrell.com

carolynbirrell.com